Stress and Health

Stress and Health

Understanding the Effects and Examining Interventions

Editor

Alyx Taylor

MDPI • Basel • Beijing • Wuhan • Barcelona • Belgrade • Manchester • Tokyo • Cluj • Tianjin

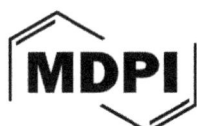

Editor
Alyx Taylor
School of Psychology,
Sport and Physical Activity,
Department of Physiology,
AECC University College
UK

Editorial Office
MDPI
St. Alban-Anlage 66
4052 Basel, Switzerland

This is a reprint of articles from the Special Issue published online in the open access journal *Healthcare* (ISSN 2227-9032) (available at: https://www.mdpi.com/journal/healthcare/special_issues/stress_health).

For citation purposes, cite each article independently as indicated on the article page online and as indicated below:

LastName, A.A.; LastName, B.B.; LastName, C.C. Article Title. *Journal Name* **Year**, *Volume Number*, Page Range.

ISBN 978-3-0365-0780-4 (Hbk)
ISBN 978-3-0365-0781-1 (PDF)

Cover image courtesy of Micah Hallahan.

© 2021 by the authors. Articles in this book are Open Access and distributed under the Creative Commons Attribution (CC BY) license, which allows users to download, copy and build upon published articles, as long as the author and publisher are properly credited, which ensures maximum dissemination and a wider impact of our publications.

The book as a whole is distributed by MDPI under the terms and conditions of the Creative Commons license CC BY-NC-ND.

Contents

About the Editor vii

Preface to "Stress and Health" ix

Ivone Castro-Vale and Davide Carvalho
The Pathways between Cortisol-Related Regulation Genes and PTSD Psychotherapy
Reprinted from: *Healthcare* **2020**, *8*, 376, doi:10.3390/healthcare8040376 1

Ivone Castro-Vale, Milton Severo, Davide Carvalho and Rui Mota-Cardoso
Vulnerability Factors Associated with Lifetime Posttraumatic Stress Disorder among Veterans
40 Years after War
Reprinted from: *Healthcare* **2020**, *8*, 359, doi:10.3390/healthcare8040359 31

Wonjung Ryu and Hyerin Yang
A Qualitative Case Study on Influencing Factors of Parents' Child Abuse of North Korean
Refugees in South Korea
Reprinted from: *Healthcare* **2021**, *9*, 49, doi:10.3390/healthcare9010049 45

Anna Sánchez-Aragón, Angel Belzunegui-Eraso and Òscar Prieto-Flores
Results of Mentoring in the Psychosocial Well-Being of Young Immigrants and Refugees in
Spain
Reprinted from: *Healthcare* **2021**, *9*, 13, doi:10.3390/healthcare9010013 57

**Yekta Said Can, Heather Iles-Smith, Niaz Chalabianloo, Deniz Ekiz, Javier
Fernández-Álvarez, Claudia Repetto, Giuseppe Riva and Cem Ersoy**
How to Relax in Stressful Situations: A Smart Stress Reduction System
Reprinted from: *Healthcare* **2020**, *8*, 100, doi:10.3390/healthcare8020100 75

About the Editor

Alyx Taylor is the Research Lead for the School of Psychology, Sport and Physical Activity and the convener for the Research Centre for Health, Exercise and Sports Science (CHESS). Dr. Taylor originally obtained her B.S. in Biochemistry and Chemistry at Queen Elizabeth College London, M.S. in Psychology at the University of Derby, and undertook her Ph.D. at Imperial College London. Dr. Taylor's research interests concern the psychology and neuroendocrinology associated with affective disorders and the human stress response. Dr. Taylor enjoys contributing to the academic community as a journal editor. Dr. Taylor is a Fellow of Advance HE and an active member of the British Association of Sport and Exercise Sciences, the Research Council Complementary Medicine, and the British Psychological Society.

Preface to "Stress and Health"

The human stress response consists of coordinated physiological changes that prepare the body for optimum cognitive processing and physical activity to meet challenges or overcome threats. Stressful stimuli can arise from work, living conditions, financial resources, personal relationships, and the physical or mental health status of the individual and their family members. Some individuals appear to manage high-stress situations without negative effects, and may even report that they thrive on high stress levels at work or in leisure activities. In contrast, others do not have the same resilience and experience negative changes to their physical and mental health. The possible effects on the mental health of service personnel were acknowledged in the last century, leading to the development of supportive services. It is also recognized that professional groups including healthcare workers, firefighters, and police can be exposed to highly stressful incidents in the course of their work, the result of which is some individuals experiencing mental health problems, including posttraumatic stress disorder, anxiety, or depression, and therefore require effective interventions. Other sources of chronic stress for specific groups of people around the world include, for example, civilians living in war zones or refugees adapting to a new environment, culture, and language. These individuals may experience posttraumatic stress disorder and difficulties with normal family relationships. Within their home country, people can experience chronic stress from situations such as domestic violence or poverty. Natural disasters such as earthquakes and floods can cause acute, long-term, or recurring hardship and stress through loss of homes, businesses, and loved ones. In these situations, individuals and different generations in their families are involved. Many individuals remain resilient, while some suffer negative effects on their mental or physical health. An individual's stress response has been shown to arise from the interaction between their genetic inheritance and the influence of their environment through epigenetic changes and other pathways. For the developing fetus, the uterus is a protective environment. However, evidence indicates that maternal experiences of intense or prolonged stress, anxiety, or depression during pregnancy may influence the developing infant [1]. On the positive side, evidence indicates that a strong sense of coherence can help mothers manage perinatal stress, which reduces the risk of depression [2], and it is possible to enhance this through intervention. Therefore, supportive perinatal interventions may benefit multiple generations of the family. In summary, the health of individuals and their children may be enhanced by interventions to help them manage the effects of stressful life experiences and environments. The papers presented here provide insights into the pathological effects of stress that may disrupt the normal relationships between individuals and their families. These papers also emphasize the need for the provision of innovative and effective interventions.

References

1. Glover, V.; O'Connor, T.G.; O'Donnell, K. Prenatal stress and the programming of the HPA axis. *Neurosci. Biobehav. Rev.* **2010**, *35*, 17–22. doi:10.1016/j.neubiorev.2009.11.008.
2. Goren, G.; Sarid, O.; Philippou, P.; Taylor, A. Sense of coherence mediates the links between job status prior to birth and postpartum depression: A structured equation modeling approach. *Int. J. Environ. Res. Public Health* **2020**, *17*, 6189. doi:10.3390/ijerph17176189

Alyx Taylor

Editor

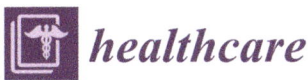

Review

The Pathways between Cortisol-Related Regulation Genes and PTSD Psychotherapy

Ivone Castro-Vale [1,2,*] and Davide Carvalho [3]

[1] Medical Psychology Unit, Department of Clinical Neurosciences and Mental Health, Faculty of Medicine, University of Porto, Al. Prof. Hernâni Monteiro, 4200-319 Porto, Portugal
[2] i3S-Institute for Research and Innovation in Health, University of Porto, Rua Alfredo Allen, 208, 4200-135 Porto, Portugal
[3] Department of Endocrinology, Diabetes and Metabolism, São João Hospital University Centre, Faculty of Medicine, University of Porto, Al. Prof. Hernâni Monteiro, 4200-319 Porto, Portugal; davideccarvalho@gmail.com
* Correspondence: ivonecastrovale@i3s.up.pt

Received: 21 August 2020; Accepted: 24 September 2020; Published: 1 October 2020

Abstract: Post-traumatic stress disorder (PTSD) only develops after exposure to a traumatic event in some individuals. PTSD can be chronic and debilitating, and is associated with co-morbidities such as depression, substance use, and cardiometabolic disorders. One of the most important pathophysiological mechanisms underlying the development of PTSD and its subsequent maintenance is a dysfunctional hypothalamic–pituitary–adrenal (HPA) axis. The corticotrophin-releasing hormone, cortisol, glucocorticoid receptor (GR), and their respective genes are some of the mediators of PTSD's pathophysiology. Several treatments are available, including medication and psychotherapies, although their success rate is limited. Some pharmacological therapies based on the HPA axis are currently being tested in clinical trials and changes in HPA axis biomarkers have been found to occur in response not only to pharmacological treatments, but also to psychotherapy—including the epigenetic modification of the GR gene. Psychotherapies are considered to be the first line treatments for PTSD in some guidelines, even though they are effective for some, but not for all patients with PTSD. This review aims to address how knowledge of the HPA axis-related genetic makeup can inform and predict the outcomes of psychotherapeutic treatments.

Keywords: posttraumatic stress disorder; psychotherapy; glucocorticoids; cortisol; glucocorticoid receptor; *NR3C1*; *FKBP5*

---

1. Introduction

Post-traumatic stress disorder (PTSD) is a trauma- and stressor-related disorder which can only develop after the experience of a major traumatic event (TE) [1]. In the fifth Edition of the Diagnostic and Statistical Manual of Mental Disorders (DSM-5) [1], PTSD criteria were redefined and are now characterised by four symptom clusters, namely: re-experience of the TE; avoidance of stimuli associated with the TE; negative cognitions and mood; and alterations in arousal, all of which must last for more than one month and cause significant clinical distress or impairment in important areas of functioning. Although the experience of TEs is very frequent in the population, with a lifetime prevalence ranging from 64–90% [2,3], only around 10% of the population will develop the disorder [4]. PTSD development is highly dependent on the type of TE, the individual genetic makeup, and other risk factors, as is also the manifestation of different symptoms and the severity of PTSD [5,6].

When an individual experiences a TE, the stress-reactive systems are activated, which include the sympathoadrenomedullary drive and the hypothalamic–pituitary–adrenal (HPA) axis [7]. Individuals with a history of previous increased vulnerability to PTSD development (e.g., childhood adversities which modify the stress-reactive systems [8,9]) can experience PTSD symptoms immediately after the TE experience, or later on, while those with no such vulnerability can develop PTSD due to specific direct TE-related effects on the stress systems (e.g., epigenetic modifications or trauma interaction with specific single nucleotide polymorphisms (SNPs)).

The reason why only a limited number of people who experienced TEs develop PTSD has been subject to debate in the scientific community [10]. Gene/environment (G × E) interactions have been indicated as reliable mechanisms [11]. Indeed, it appears that vulnerability to develop PTSD can result from exposure to environmental adversity in cases of specific genetic makeup, such as, for example, SNPs and the epigenome [12]. TEs can also influence genetic expression through epigenetic mechanisms. Furthermore, exposure to other previous adverse experiences increases the risk of PTSD development [13], through epigenetic mechanisms [8]. SNPs can also interact with environmental exposure and epigenetic modifications to increase the risk of PTSD development [14].

A recent systematic review found that the examination of all the included PTSD studies consistently implicated DNA methylation and gene expression changes in the HPA axis and inflammatory genes in PTSD pathophysiology [15]. Indeed, genetic factors have been estimated to account for 30–46% of the variance in PTSD [16,17]. Being a stress-related disorder, HPA axis regulator genes have been extensively studied—such as the glucocorticoid receptor (GR) and FK506 binding protein 51 (FKBP5) genes [10]. Although the risk of developing PTSD is polygenetic, a recent meta-analysis found SNPs in these two genes to be associated with PTSD [18]. Furthermore, the GR gene (*NR3C1*) has been considered to be a candidate gene which underlies the neurobiological-related glucocorticoid (GC) processes involved in the development or maintenance of PTSD [12].

PTSD is a heterogeneous disorder and the determinants of different conditional risks for PTSD development can be categorised in several ways [19], including the type and burden of the TE and the sex and age of the exposed subject, which also determine the symptomatic expression, clinical trajectories, co-morbidity, and treatment response. Furthermore, the HPA axis regulation of the response to TE and stress is highly complex and is subject to a large degree of variability.

As a result, different clinical trajectories of PTSD development have been described in different trauma-exposed populations [10,20–23]. The longer-lasting prospective study found five classes of trajectories based on PTSD symptom severity, which were assessed using the Clinician-Administered PTSD Scale score, during the six years after traumatic injury. These are: chronic (4%), recovery (6%), worsening/recovery (8%), worsening (10%), and resilient (73%) [21]. In addition, PTSD can be very debilitating and is also associated with mental and somatic comorbidity [24,25], such as depression, substance use disorders, cardiovascular conditions, and endocrine and metabolic disorders, as well as with intergenerational transmission of depression, emotion dysregulation, and HPA axis dysfunction [26–28].

Several treatments have been indicated for patients with PTSD, which mainly include pharmacotherapy and psychotherapy. As pharmacotherapy approaches have considerable high rates of non-response, significant investment has been carried out in applying other therapies—particularly psychotherapies. Various psychotherapies have been indicated for the treatment of PTSD, with reported success being superior to that of the prescription of medication in several studies [29], although their effectiveness has been questioned [30]. Accordingly, there is a need to improve existing PTSD psychotherapeutic treatments, as almost two-thirds of patients receiving prolonged exposure therapy (PE) or cognitive processing therapy (CPT)—which are the two most widely-recommended first-line therapies—maintained the same diagnosis posttreatment [31].

It is becoming clearer that psychotherapeutic interventions must be individually tailored. Psychotherapeutic intervention in patients with PTSD has been associated with change in plasma cortisol [32], and more recently with changes in the epigenome [33,34]. Furthermore, SNPs in the GR and *FKBP5* genes and *FKBP5* epigenomic alterations predict psychotherapeutic outcomes [33,35,36]. Another ten genes, including a gene related with stress vulnerability (*ZFP57*), have also been recently associated with psychotherapeutic outcomes in a longitudinal study of genome-wide DNA methylation levels [34]. Successful treatment of PTSD patients with psychotherapy was accompanied by changes in DNA methylation.

In this paper we aim to review the extant knowledge regarding the interplay between the HPA axis regulatory genes and psychotherapeutic interventions for patients with PTSD, by taking into account the previously-reported HPA axis-related G × E interactions involved in PTSD pathophysiology, as well as the interactions between the genetic makeup and psychotherapy and the urgent need to improve patients' psychotherapeutic outcomes.

2. The HPA Axis

2.1. Neuroendocrine Regulation

The HPA axis is necessary for adaptation to stress. Physiological stimuli and stress activate the HPA axis (a three-organ hormonal cascade and feedback cycle) which leads to GC (cortisol in humans) secretion and release from the adrenal cortex (Box 1). Indeed, cortisol is both the primary GC which signals the stress response and the primary inhibitor of continuing HPA axis activity and of the autonomic stress responses [7].

Box 1. The hypothalamic–pituitary–adrenal (HPA) axis.

Both physiological stimuli and stress trigger the HPA axis leading to glucocorticoids (GCs, cortisol in humans) release from the adrenal cortex:

- Physiological homeostatic challenges involve, through sensory relays, the direct noradrenergic and peptidergic (originating mainly from the nucleus of the solitary tract) stimulation of the corticotrophin-releasing hormone (CRH) neurons which are located in the dorsomedial parvocellular (mp) division of the hypothalamic paraventricular nucleus (PVN) [37]. Further processing of the information includes glutamatergic, serotoninergic, and cytokine stimulation of the PVN. Under specific conditions, GABA can also stimulate the HPA axis at the PVN.
- Anticipatory responses involve the trans-synaptic activation of the HPA axis through the integration of multimodal sensory information, and the respective higher processing, which involves the ventral hippocampus, the medial prefrontal cortex, and the amygdala, among other limbic structures [7].
- Hypothalamic PVN is subject to regulation by several structures by way of glutamatergic and GABAergic neurons and the endocannabinoid system.
- The amygdala plays an important role in the defensive responses to learned threats. [38]. The lateral nucleus is important for the acquisition of aversive learning [39,40]. The aversive stimulus is recognised and processed in the amygdala's basolateral complex, which connects with the central nucleus to stimulate the brainstem through CRH projections to the locus coeruleus [41] and the hypothalamus preparing the person to cope with the stimulus.
- GCs act through rapid non-genomic mechanisms in the basolateral amygdala through a membrane GC receptor (mGR), inducing the release of endocannabinoids from postsynaptic membranes, generating a retrograde feedback suppression on GABAergic neurons, and thereby driving the release of norepinephrine to the amygdala, which is required for emotional memory acquisition [42,43]. The prefrontal cortex and the hippocampus project to both the PVN and the amygdala in order to regulate the response to the aversive stimulus [7,44].
- CRH binds to the CRH type 1 receptor in the anterior pituitary, stimulating the release of the adrenocorticotrophic hormone (ACTH) into the bloodstream. Arginine vasopressin is co-released and it complements CRH actions in ACTH release.
- ACTH action on the adrenal cortex leads to cortisol production and release, which is potentiated by the sympathetic nervous system and cytokines.
- The GC response depends on the timing of the stressful event: if this event occurs during the ascending phase of the ultradian pulse, it tends to have a greater level of response than if it were to occur during the falling phase [7,45].
- Cortisol serves several functions, including mobilisation of energy to cope with the aversive stimuli, memory processing, immune system modulation, the termination of the response by active feedback processes, repressing all unnecessary activity—such as growth (emergency mode: when a person is faced with a traumatic event (TE) GCs inactivate all non-essential activities for survival [46]). Another important effect of GCs is to enhance the consolidation of the memories of fear and other strong emotions to facilitate coping with re-exposure [47].

Cortisol exerts crucial feedback effects on binding to GRs in the hypothalamus and the pituitary, which reduces the release of both corticotrophin-releasing hormone (CRH) and adrenocorticotrophic hormone (ACTH) [7]. GC-bound mGR releases endocannabinoids, which, in turn, inhibit the release of glutamate, which reduces the stimulation of the hypothalamic paraventricular nucleus (PVN) CRH neurons. GABAergic and neuropeptidergic inputs also play important roles in inhibiting CRH release. Transsynaptic GR mediated HPA axis inhibition also occurs in the hippocampus, as well as the prefrontal cortex and the hindbrain. These feedback effects are very important to stop the exposure to the catabolic actions of GC and the sympathetic nervous system effects. Norepinephrine is an important mediator of the central nervous system (CNS) and autonomic stress responses. Norepinephrine and CRH interact in the hypothalamus, locus coeruleus, and amygdala circuit, integrating autonomic and HPA axis responses to stress.

The HPA axis regulation is highly complex. In addition to trans-synaptic regulation, the secretion of CRH by the PVN is also regulated by GCs, arginine vasopressin, and oxytocin [48]. The secretion of ACTH is regulated by GCs. The sensitivity of the adrenal cortex to ACTH is another possible limiting step in HPA axis activity. For in the serum, cortisol is bound to proteins—mainly corticosteroid-binding globulin (CBG)—where only 5% of systemic cortisol is free and bioactive (Figure 1) [49]. The availability of CBG, which is negatively regulated by GC, is another influence on GC actions. At the cellular level, cortisol availability is regulated by tissue-specific enzymes, as well as the 11β-hydroxysteroid dehydrogenases (11β-HSDs). 11βHSD-1 is widely expressed in all the GC target tissues (e.g., neurons and glial cells), where it converts cortisone to active cortisol, whereas 11βHSD-2 has the opposite effect, particularly in the kidney (Figure 1) [50]. At the cellular level, cortisol actions are also regulated by the GR and its respective *NR3C1* gene, as well as co-chaperones of the GR, such as FKBP5, among others.

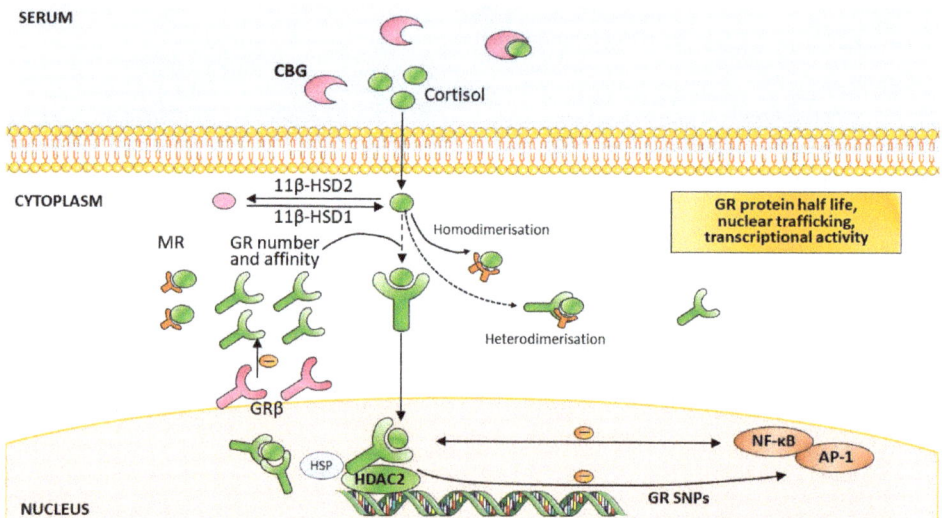

Figure 1. Modulators of the cellular action of glucocorticoids. These modulators include glucocorticoid availability, glucocorticoid receptor number and affinity, GRβ isoform expression, glucocorticoid receptor signalling, mineralocorticoid receptor signalling, glucocorticoid receptor–gene interaction, and glucocorticoid receptor single nucleotide polymorphisms. Abbreviations: 11β-HSD: 11-β-hydroxysteroid dehydrogenase; CBG: Corticosteroid-binding globulin; GR: glucocorticoid receptor; HSP: heat shock protein; MR: mineralocorticoid receptor; NF-κB: nuclear factor k B; SNPs: single nucleotide polymorphisms; HDAC2: histone deacetylase 2; AP-1: activator protein 1. Adapted by permission from [Nature] [51].

Cortisol alone, therefore, cannot be considered to reflect the HPA axis regulation of the stress response. Furthermore, cortisol response to stressful events is moderated by sex—with women showing greater variability in the HPA axis response than men [52,53]. Testosterone has been shown to inhibit the stress response, whereas in women, estradiol has an important moderating role in the activation of the HPA axis in response to stress [7]. HPA axis stress response is also moderated by the stage of development and the age of the subject, as well as the type, intensity, and duration of the stressful event. Additionally, also important to mention is the fact that cortisol is difficult to measure accurately to represent the reflection of HPA axis activity, as most methods show considerable intraindividual variability and, as described above, HPA axis function depends on a great variety of factors [54].

2.2. The GC Receptors

The HPA axis—through the secretion of cortisol—is the primary hormonal mediator of stress responses (Box 1). GC actions are mediated by two types of receptors: the mineralocorticoid receptor (MR) and the GR. The MR has a 6–10-fold higher affinity for binding GCs than the GR [55]. The MR is basally occupied, while the GR is only activated during periods of stress and during the circadian peak of the HPA axis activity. The MR is important in terms of the time of day of HPA axis activity and the regulation of basal circadian and ultradian rhythms. Whereas the GR is widely found in the brain, the MR is restricted to the limbic areas [7]. The capability to cope with a TE depends on the balance of these two receptors in the regulation of the stress response [56] as low GC concentrations enhance MR homodimerisation, while GC stress levels induce MR–GR heterodimerisation [57]. The MR has a role in the appraisal of the threat and initiation of the response (Figure 1) [56].

The GR has three domains: the N-terminal transactivating domain (NTD), the DNA binding domain (DBD) (which binds to DNA GC response elements (GRE)), and the C-terminal ligand-binding domain (LBD) [58]. The NTD is the most variable domain, due to alternative translation initiation. There are many GR isoforms which depend on alternative splicing at several points of the *NR3C1* gene. Alternative translation initiation and post-translational modifications add to the functional pool of GC signalling diversity—which has tissue and cell specificity [59,60]. Epigenetic mechanisms which regulate gene transcription and expression have differential functional effects depending both on the gene's region where they occur and on the SNPs' makeup [61]. In addition, the location of the SNPs has specific influences on gene function [62].

The unbound GR is not alone in the cell's cytoplasm, as it is associated with a multiprotein complex, including chaperone proteins and immunophilins [63]. Upon GC binding, this complex conformation changes and the GR becomes hyperphosphorylated and translocates to the nucleus, where it regulates the transcription of various genes directly and indirectly [46]. The GR binds to GRE as a homodimer directing transactivation of target genes. GC-induced gene expression is frequently cell type-specific, which has been shown to be dependent on the accessibility of the GR-binding site. In turn, this is determined by the chromatin structure and DNA methylation, as well as histone acetylation and methylation (HDAC2) (Figure 1) [58]. Bound-GRs also act as monomers, by interacting with other transcription factors, such as activator protein 1 (AP-1) and nuclear factor k (NF-kB), which represses their transcriptional activity and results in less pro-inflammatory effects (Figure 1) [64].

Furthermore, GCs have fast acting non-genomic actions which are mediated by cytosolic GRs and mGRs and use the activity of various kinases, thus adding greater complexity to GC signalling [65]. The effects are strongly dependent on both cell type and the cellular context. The existence of mGRs in the neuronal cells of the hypothalamus, basolateral amygdala, and hippocampus [42] plays an important role in rapid energy mobilisation and memory consolidation under stress, as well as rapidly preparing the cell for the ultimate genomic effects [66,67].

Chaperones and co-chaperones influence GR affinity for GCs. In particular, the co-chaperone of the heat shock protein (hsp)-90 *FKBP5* gene is subject to the transcriptional influence of the GR upon cortisol binding, leading to an increase in its expression, which is associated with GC resistance, serving as an intracellular feedback control of GC actions [68,69].

2.3. GR Gene and Other Genes that Regulate the HPA Axis

The most-studied gene related to the HPA axis is the GR *NR3C1* gene, which is located on chromosome 5q31-32 and is a member of the nuclear hormone receptor superfamily of ligand-activated transcription factors [70]. The human GR gene has nine exons, whereas exon 9 alternative splicing generates two GR isoforms: GRα and GRβ. The first exon is in effect a set of nine exons, which are referred to as A–J (excluding "G"), which are not translated and result in different mRNA, as they are independently controlled by a unique promoter which is located immediately upstream and thus influences the translation start site [71,72]. In the 5′ untranslated region of the *NR3C1* gene, there is a cytosine–phosphate–guanine dinucleotides (CpG) island which includes seven of the first exon's set of nine exons: 1_D, 1_J, 1_E, 1_B, 1_F, 1_C and 1_H [71] and is a target of DNA differential methylation studies.

Several functional SNPs (Table 1) of the *NR3C1* gene have been extensively studied, namely: TthIIII, ER22/23EK, N363S, BclI, and GR-9β [73].

Table 1. Single nucleotide polymorphisms (SNPs) of the *NR3C1*, *FKBP5*, and *CRHR1* genes which have been associated with post-traumatic stress disorder (PTSD) or which have altered sensitivity of the hypothalamus–pituitary–adrenal axis.

Gene	SNP Custom Name	dbSNP ID	Wild Allele	Variant Allele	GR Sensitivity *
NR3C1	TthIIII	rs10052957	C	T	↓ †
	ER22/23EK	rs6189/rs6190	G/G	A/A	↓
	N363S	rs6195 (rs56149945) ‡	A	G	↑
	BclI	rs41423247	C	G	↑
	GR-9β (A3669G) ¥	rs6198	A	G	↓
		rs258747	A	G	?
		rs10482612	G	A	↓
		rs6191	C	A	↓
	NR3C1-1	rs10482605	T	C	↓
FKBP5		rs3800373	A	C	↓
		rs9296158	G	A	↓
		rs1360780	C	T	↓
		rs9470080	C	T	↓
CRHR1		rs110402	G	A	↓
		rs242924	G	T	?
		rs12944712	G	A	?
		rs12938031	A	G	?
		rs4792887	C	T	?

* Studied specifically for GR sensitivity or inferred from functional research. † Only with the ER22/23EK; ↑: GR hypersensitivity; ↓: GR resistance; ?: unknown. ‡ Aliases. ¥ Also known as. Abbreviation: dbSNP ID: Single Nucleotide Polymorphism Database identification. Adapted by permission from [10].

The TthIIII SNP (rs10052957) is a C to T change in the promoter of the GR gene, and is only functional when associated with ER22/23EK [74].

The ER22/23EK polymorphism (rs6189/rs6190) is located in the transactivation domain and results in altered translation to the GR protein: glutamic acid-arginine (E-R) to glutamic acid-lysine (E-K) [75]. This SNP has been associated with relative GC resistance [76,77], which in turn has been attributed to the reduced transactivating capacity of the GR [78].

The N363S SNP (rs6195; alias rs56149945) results from one nucleotide substitution in codon 363 of exon 2, and the subsequent alteration from asparagine (N) to serine (S) [75]. This SNP is associated with increased sensitivity to GCs in vivo, which was manifested by significantly enhanced suppression of serum cortisol levels after a low dose of dexamethasone [79], which is probably due to increased transactivating capacity [10,76].

The *BclI* intronic SNP (rs41423247) which is situated downstream of exon 2, results from a C to G substitution at nucleotide 646, and has been associated with increased sensitivity to GCs [80,81]. This SNP was associated with emotional memory performance in healthy individuals [82], although its action mechanism is not known [10,73].

The 9β (also referred to as A3669G) SNP (rs6198) which consists of a naturally-occurring A to G substitution in the 3' UTR of exon 9β [73], is associated with increased expression and stability of the GRβ isoform of the GR [62], and with GC resistance, probably owing to decreased transrepression [10,83,84].

Other SNPs of the GR gene are associated with PTSD and depression, such as: rs258747 [18,85], rs10482612 [86], rs6191, rs33388 [87], rs6196, and rs10482605 [88].

The *FKBP5* gene, which is located in the human chromosome 6p21.31 [89], has also been extensively studied as it encodes a co-chaperone of hsp-90 in the GR molecular complex, which influences cortisol binding and subsequent conformational changes in the GR and the subsequent translocation to the nucleus [10]. FKBP5 is implicated in the feedback regulation of the GC response, as GCs increase *FKBP5* expression, which in turn decreases GR affinity for GCs. This is considered to be the ultra-short negative feedback loop for GR activity [90,91].

FKBP5 overexpression is associated with GC resistance [68,69]. This increase in GC resistance has not been associated with higher plasma cortisol levels [92]. Four functional SNPs (Table 1) in the *FKBP5* gene (rs9296158, rs3800373, rs1360780, and rs9470080) have been identified which are associated with GR resistance, in normal, mainly Afro-descent individuals (Figure 2) [93].

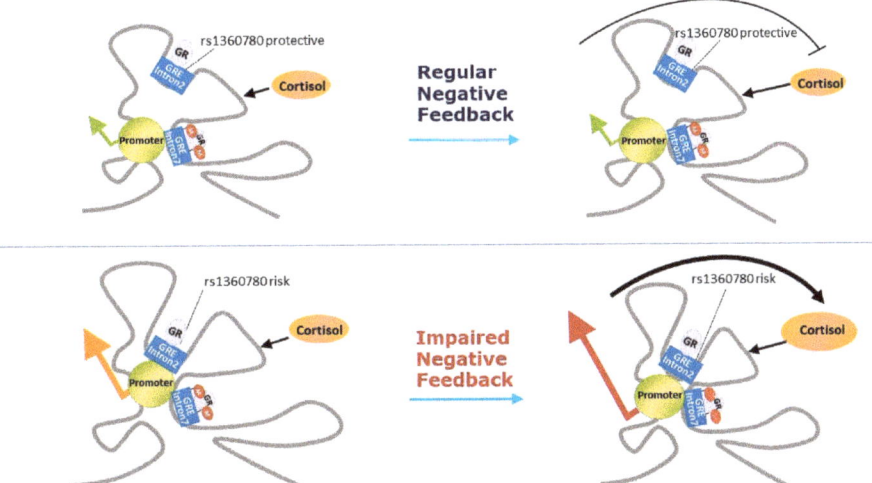

Figure 2. Representation of the epigenetic modification in *FKBP5*. The single-nucleotide polymorphism rs1360780 which is close to a functional GRE in intron 2 constitutes the genetic predisposition for an increased *FKBP5* transcriptional response to stress. Demethylation with higher cortisol levels is possibly restricted to certain developmental periods (e.g., childhood). The exposure to childhood trauma leads to an increased activation of *FKBP5* due to a reduction in DNA methylation in SNP risk allele carriers. Adapted by permission from [Nature] [94].

The corticotrophin-releasing hormone receptor 1 (*CRHR1*) and 2 (*CRHR2*) genes have also been studied. In addition, variants for *CRHR1* (Table 1), rs110402, rs242924, rs7209436, rs12944712, rs12938031, and rs4792887 have been studied [93,95,96] and some of them demonstrate G × E interactions [97,98].

2.4. Epigenetic Regulation of the HPA Axis

Epigenetics refers to modifiable, potentially heritable, non-nucleotide changes to DNA transcription which are essential for normal cell differentiation and neurogenesis [99]. These changes can both be stable over time and dynamically responsive to environmental challenges such as nutritional, pharmacological, physical, and psychosocial changes, providing experience-dependent DNA modulation. Three main mechanisms have been identified for epigenetic gene transcription regulation and expression. The first is the DNA methylation of the cytosine pyrimidine ring of CpG sites, which suppresses gene transcription. It should be noted that these dinucleotides are especially numerous in the promoter regions (CpG islands). However, DNA methylation of the gene body can have the opposite effect [100]. The second mechanism consists of post-translational modifications of histone proteins, such as methylation, phosphorylation, and acetylation, which alter DNA that bind to regulatory proteins as well as the availability of chromatin for transcriptional activity. The third mechanism comprises RNAs (including siRNAs, miRNAs, and piRNAs) and long noncoding RNAs, which also regulate gene expression [99,101–104].

These modifications constitute the epigenome, which can record long-lasting influences from the environment and can be inherited [105,106]. These influences from the environment can occur at specific sensitive periods of development, including exposures in adulthood. DNA methylation is the most studied epigenetic mechanism of genes involved in HPA axis regulation, such as *NR3C1* and *FKBP5*. In particular, methylation of *NR3C1* is thought to underlie the programming of the HPA axis function in response to environmental exposures, such as childhood abuse [107,108]. Furthermore, higher cortisol levels demethylate *FKBP5* intron 7 in carriers of the SNP rs1360780 T risk allele possibly in specific developmental periods such as childhood, increasing *FKBP5* expression and GR resistance [94].

A review of the methylation effects on the GR gene concluded that early life adversity has been repeatedly shown to be associated with hypermethylation of the non-coding first exons [71], which could impair HPA axis functioning, specifically with the respective decreased GR expression, and predispose the exposed subjects to several psychiatric disorders.

The noncoding RNAs epigenetic mechanism has also been shown to influence the regulation of the HPA axis in response to stress. The miRNA miR-320a interacts with the *FKBP5* SNP rs3800373 C risk allele, leading to increased *FKBP5* expression and GR resistance [109]. Other studies of noncoding RNAs influences on the HPA axis regulation are reviewed elsewhere [110].

In sum, the HPA axis response to stress challenges has multiple levels of regulation which are influenced by variability in genes (SNPs) and epigenome. These effects can further expand environmental influences on genetic expression and consequently on endophenotypes and phenotypes [14]. This means that nature and nurture interactions have endless possibilities. This phenomenon can also be viewed from a therapeutic point-of-view, as these interactions can use pharmacotherapy and psychotherapy to environmentally manipulate these genes—by gene, by epigenome, and by environment interactions.

3. HPA Axis and PTSD

As the new DSM-5 classification rightfully implies, PTSD is a disorder of the stress adaptation system, which is initiated by the influence of the TE on a susceptible person [111]. Accordingly, HPA axis dysfunction has been consistently pointed out to constitute the main pathophysiologic mechanism involved in the development and maintenance of PTSD [54,112,113].

Although PTSD only develops after exposure to TEs, other risk factors exist which increase the probability of a TE influencing the development of PTSD [4,6]. Some of these risk factors also influence the HPA axis function, examples being childhood adversity, parental PTSD, or the occurrence of prior TE or PTSD [9,28]. Exposure to these TEs generates anticipatory responses of the HPA axis, which in turn are moderated by SNPs and the epigenome [7,54,114]. Another important moderator between HPA axis functioning and PTSD is the biological sex, even when controlling for confounders. It is well known that women have a greater risk of developing PTSD than men [115,116]. Interestingly, female victims of sexual assault with lower hippocampal volumes showed increased risk of developing PTSD [117].

The most studied regulator of the HPA axis in PTSD is the GR [10]. Patients with PTSD show reduced GC signalling, which has been shown to be associated with increased GR responsiveness or sensitivity [113]. Indeed, hypersensitivity of the GR in PTSD patients has been found in several studies [111,118–121] and has been specifically attributed to decreased GC signalling [113]. In addition, studies which assess learning and memory also argue that PTSD patients have increased CNS GC hypersensitivity [122]. Indeed, cortisol plays an important role in coping with the emotional memories of trauma by enhancing consolidation and by decreasing retrieval and working memory [42].

Accordingly, lower cortisol levels in saliva, blood, or urine have been found in two metanalyses [118,123] in specific samples and assessment moments of the day, although lower cortisol levels were also found to be associated with trauma exposure, especially in the afternoon and evening. Another metanalysis, which included only saliva samples, showed that morning cortisol levels were significantly lower in PTSD patients when compared to controls [124]. Accordingly, a recent metanalysis found lower concentrations of 24-h urinary cortisol in PTSD patients when compared to controls [125]. Furthermore, neurobiological correlates of PTSD symptom clusters have also been found in some studies to show a negative association between cortisol levels and specific symptom clusters, such as intrusion, avoidance, and numbing e.g., [126,127].

On the other hand, CRH overactivity has been pointed out to be a possible model of HPA axis dysfunction in PTSD [54]. Central spinal fluid CRH levels have been found to be increased in patients with PTSD [128–130]. This finding is consistent with decreased GC signalling in PTSD, as GCs are potent inhibitors of CRH release [131]. Consistent with these HPA axis alterations is the concept that PTSD is a fear disorder, characterised by an excessively strong learning of trauma-related fear, or a failure over time to extinguish memories of previous trauma-related fear experiences [132].

Whether these HPA axis alterations are a cause or a consequence of PTSD development, or whether they are TE exposure-related has been a matter of debate in the scientific community [54]. HPA axis-related pre-trauma altered functions have been found to be more consistently associated with PTSD. High pre-deployment GR number, low *FKBP5* mRNA expression, and high glucocorticoid-induced leucine zipper (GILZ) gene mRNA expression are all independently associated with increased risk for a high level of PTSD symptoms six months after deployment to a combat zone [133]. Accordingly, lower hair cortisol concentrations prior to deployment were associated with post-deployment PTSD symptoms related to new stressors [134]. Furthermore, different clinical trajectories after experiencing a TE are also predicted by cortisol secretion as a response to experimental stress challenges, showing lower saliva cortisol change. When assessed prior to exposure to TEs, these trajectories are less-favourable on the whole [134,135]. With regards to peritraumatic HPA axis-related risk factors, lower cortisol levels [121,136] have been found to predict PTSD development, although a metanalysis only found that heart rate was correlated with posterior PTSD symptoms, among the other biological markers studied, including cortisol measured immediately after TE [137].

Imaging studies also link PTSD pathophysiology with the HPA axis. As an example, lower levels of expression of *FKBP5* were associated with smaller hippocampus and medial orbitofrontal cortex in PTSD patients when compared to non-PTSD controls [138]. A systematic review has shown that lower hippocampal volumes are associated with PTSD [139]. Excessive activation of the amygdala on exposure to threat stimuli has also been demonstrated in patients with PTSD [140].

3.1. PTSD and GC Regulation Genes SNPs

Genome wide association studies have failed to find associations between HPA axis-related genes and PTSD e.g., [141]. However, a recent meta-analysis found that SNPs in *NR3C1* and *FKBP5* genes (rs258747 in *NR3C1* and rs9296158 in *FKBP5*) are significantly associated with PTSD [18]. It has been hypothesised that some of the SNPs of the *NR3C1* gene associated with PTSD could be in linkage disequilibrium with previously-identified functional SNPs [85]. With regards *FKBP5*, the risk allele of the SNP rs9296158 has been previously associated with GR resistance in normal Afro-descent individuals and with GR hypersensitivity in PTSD patients (Figure 2) [93].

Although no main effects had been found for any of the previously-identified functional GR gene SNPs in PTSD, the severity of PTSD symptoms and basal plasma cortisol levels were negatively correlated within war veterans with PTSD who are homozygous for the BclI SNP. In this same subgroup of PTSD patients, the authors also found a tendency for an increased response to a test of peripheral GC sensitivity which correlated with higher PTSD symptoms [142]. In cardiac surgery patients, homozygous carriers of the BclI SNP variant allele showed significantly lower preoperative plasma cortisol levels and more traumatic memories six months after surgery and intensive care unit treatment [143]. A significant interaction effect was found of haplotype BclI carrier state and childhood trauma on the pre-deployment GR number [133]. In this study, childhood trauma and a pre-deployment high GR number both predicted the subsequent development of a high level of PTSD symptoms. The higher GR number in the PTSD group was maintained after one and six months [10,144].

With regards *FKBP5*, the four functional SNPs which have been identified as being associated with GR resistance in normal, mainly Afro-descent individuals (rs9296158, rs3800373, rs1360780, and rs9470080) have all shown hypersensitivity to GC in patients with PTSD (Figure 2) [10,93]. This finding suggests that other factors influence the functionality of these SNPs. Interestingly, in this study, these SNPs significantly interacted with the severity of child abuse to predict levels of adult PTSD symptoms [93]. In a study on the genetics of substance dependence which also screened for PTSD, the *FKBP5* rs9470080 genotype (TT) was shown to moderate PTSD risk in interaction with childhood abuse in Afro–American participants, but not in the case of European–Americans [145]. Afro–Americans who were carriers of the TT genotype, but with no experience of childhood adversity, demonstrate the lowest risk for PTSD, but inversely they had the highest level if they had experienced childhood adversity. This result suggests that childhood adversity changes *FKBP5* gene functionality, as was the case in the study by Binder et al. [93]. A study of gene expression in 15 patients with PTSD, comparing them with 20 participants without PTSD, all of whom had been exposed to the World Trade Centre attacks, found that *FKBP5* expression was significantly reduced in current PTSD which was predicted by cortisol when entered with PTSD symptom severity in a regression analysis [146]. This study was extended to include SNP analyses of the *FKBP5* gene, as well as a sample of recovered PTSD patients and it was found that any of the four PTSD risk-related SNPs was a negative predictor of *FKBP5* expression, which in turn was related to lower levels of plasma cortisol and higher PTSD symptom severity [147]. Low pre-deployment levels of *FKBP5* mRNA expression were independently associated with the increased risk of high PTSD symptoms when assessed six months after deployment [148]. However, the study found no associations between *FKBP5* SNPs rs1360780 and rs3800373 haplotypes and pre-deployment *FKBP5* mRNA expression or GR number. On the other hand, in a sample of 412 chronic pain outpatients, the *FKBP5* gene SNP rs9470080 was associated with lifetime PTSD and it was found that participants without the risk allele had decreased PTSD risk, even in the presence of high levels of previous trauma exposure [149]. The interaction of genotype and PTSD symptoms associated with specific gene expression patterns suggested the existence of different biological PTSD endophenotypes, which are determined by functional SNPs in the *FKBP5* gene [150]. In this study, PTSD patients carrying the risk allele of the *FKBP5* gene SNP rs9296158 showed GR super-sensitivity with the dexamethasone suppression test, whereas those without the risk allele had lower baseline serum cortisol concentrations. PTSD carriers of this SNP risk allele had lower *FKBP5* mRNA expression, whilst those without PTSD had increased expression. However, in a study of 3890 US service members deployed to Iraq and Afghanistan, the carriers of the most frequent haplotype AGCC tended to have probable PTSD. Furthermore, each wild type variant SNP was associated with probable PTSD. In this study, the authors considered that *FKBP5* could be a risk factor for PTSD. No interactions with lifetime stressful events were found [151].

Klengel et al. [14] found that this diversity is determined by developmental impacts, such as early childhood adversities, which occurred by way of epigenetic mechanisms in the *FKBP5* SNP rs1360780

(Figure 2). This study showed that being a carrier of this *FKBP5* SNP risk allele, together with being exposed to early childhood adversities, both lead to *FKBP5* intron 7 demethylation. Furthermore, a recent meta-analysis found strong evidence of interactions between *FKBP5* genotypes in three SNPs (namely risk allele carriers of the rs1360780, rs3800373, or rs9470080) and early-life stress, which the authors considered could constitute significant risk factors for stress-related disorders such as PTSD [152]. Unfortunately, rs9296158 *FKBP5* SNP, which has been found to be associated with PTSD in a recent metanalysis [18], was not included.

The first study of the associations between *CRHR1* gene and PTSD in adults found that the SNPs rs12938031 and rs4792887 major alleles were associated with post-hurricane PTSD symptoms and that the former was also associated with PTSD diagnosis [96]. A longitudinal study of pediatric injury patients found an association of the *CRHR1* gene SNP rs12944712 with acute PTSD symptoms and their trajectory over time. Results from this study were considered preliminary, as the sample size was small [95]. One study identified that two SNPs (rs8192496 and rs2190242) in the *CRHR2* gene reduced PTSD risk among trauma-exposed female veterans. The minor allele of these SNPs was associated with reduced risk and severity of PTSD symptoms, although these findings have not been replicated [153].

The studies reviewed in this section show that GC regulation genes' SNPs have an important role in PTSD risk and development. Studies have a greater focus on *FKBP5* gene variation, and on the whole, the literature shows that SNP alleles which are associated with HPA axis hypersensitivity are associated with PTSD. G × E interactions have also been shown, particularly in cases with experience of childhood adversity.

3.2. PTSD and Epigenetic Effects

The *NR3C1*, *FKBP5*, and *CRHR1* genes methylation have all been shown to be associated with childhood adversity [8,14,108,154]. These modifications could constitute risk factors for PTSD development upon later exposure to a TE. Epigenetic modifications could also result from TE proper exposure and influence the pathophysiology of PTSD development. Methylation levels of *NR3C1* and *FKBP5* have been repeatedly associated with the status of PTSD diagnosis [155].

Despite the different methodologies across studies, a recent systematic review found strong evidence of an association between *NR3C1* increased methylation levels and decreased gene expression, which suggests a role for this gene's methylation in stress-related psychopathology [156]. Methylation levels of the *NR3C1* gene have been studied in the promoter regions of exons 1_B, 1_C, and 1_F, which are rich CpG sites. Hypermethylation of 1_F is associated with a decreased expression of the gene and accordingly with GR resistance [108]. An association between the demethylation of the GR gene exon 1_F promoter and both PTSD and plasma cortisol decline on the dexamethasone suppression test was found [157]. In this study, war-related PTSD male subjects showed greater cortisol suppression after the administration of dexamethasone, and higher levels of peripheral blood mononuclear cell lysozyme inhibition in the lysozyme suppression test. Accordingly, another study of survivors of the Rwanda genocide found that the sex-dependent salivary GR gene exon 1_F promotor DNA methylation was associated with PTSD [158]. Male but not female survivors with increased GR gene exon 1_F promotor methylation, which was associated with lower *NR3C1* expression, showed less intrusive memory of the traumatic event and reduced PTSD risk. In these studies, it was not possible to distinguish the effects of trauma from the effects of PTSD. Another study focussing on female victims of the same Rwanda Tutsi genocide, found higher peripheral blood leukocytes *NR3C1* exon 1_F promotor methylation levels than those of Tutsi non-victims [159]. However, the association between PTSD and *NR3C1* gene exon 1_F promotor methylation levels was not addressed, and in this case, hypermethylation could be attributed to trauma exposure. *NR3C1* exon 1_F promotor methylation levels negatively correlated both with cortisol levels and *NR3C1* mRNA expression levels. In this same study, those exposed to trauma showed higher methylation of CpGs located within the *NR3C2* coding sequence than non-exposed subjects. On the other hand, peripheral T lymphocytes *NR3C1* 1_B and 1_C promoters' methylation levels were found to be lower in subjects with lifetime PTSD related to different types of trauma, when compared with non-traumatised controls. Cortisol levels were inversely correlated with *NR3C1* 1_B mRNA expression. Furthermore, overall and CpG site-specific methylation levels were inversely correlated with total *NR3C1* and 1_B mRNA expression [160]. However, in this study, the *NR3C1* exon 1_F promotor methylation did not associate with PTSD risk. Another study of female interpersonal violence victims found PTSD severity to be negatively correlated with the mean percentage of *NR3C1* exon 1_F methylation [161].

FKBP5 methylation has also been extensively studied. Klengel et al. [14] found that being a carrier of the *FKBP5* SNP rs1360780 risk allele T and also being exposed to early life trauma lead to *FKBP5* intron 7 demethylation. *FKBP5* intron 7 is situated in a GC response element zone, which is subject to the action of GCs as part of the ultra-short feedback loop between FKBP5 and the GR, which leads to GR resistance, as demethylation increases levels of this co-chaperone. However, [162] no main effects of PTSD diagnosis on *FKBP5* intron 7 methylation were found in a sample of Holocaust survivors, nor in their offspring and comparison subjects. A recent study did find significantly higher intron 7 methylation levels among veterans with PTSD carrying the rs1360780 risk allele when they were compared to the non-PTSD group [163]. On the other hand, *FKBP5* exon 1 promoter methylation was associated with lower plasma cortisol levels in subjects with combat-related PTSD [33], which supports previous findings of lower *FKBP5* expression in PTSD [146].

In the case of GILZ—which is a transcription factor that is up-regulated by GC action [46]—mRNA levels were associated with PTSD in males, and were negatively associated with the methylation of the respective gene. Furthermore, the number of TEs correlated negatively with *GILZ* mRNA levels, and positively with the percentage methylation of *GILZ* just in the case of males [164].

Other approaches to the epigenomic study of PTSD pathophysiology are still being carried out. A longitudinal study of combat-related PTSD found decreases in DNA methylation in three novel genomic regions (*ZFP57*, *RNF39* and *HIST1H2APS2*) across the period of exposure which constituted marks of susceptibility to PTSD [165]. Noncoding RNAs have also been implicated in the relationship between stress and GCs and these could prove to be useful biomarkers to facilitate the prescription of personalised medicines for trauma-related disorders, as the majority of PTSD blood based microRNA studies report reduced expression in PTSD [110].

Differences in gene expression can reflect epigenetic modifications and/or interactions with SNPs. Changes in gene expression have been found to occur after combat exposure [166]. However, no longitudinal studies have examined the combination of DNA methylation and gene expression—which limits our understanding of associated TE exposure DNA methylation on gene expression [166].

The epigenetic regulation of gene expression is very much cell-type specific [112]. The previous studies researched methylation in non-CNS cells, and therefore we are unable to conclude on the neuronal methylation status, although this could well reflect exposure to environmental influences [100], as has been shown for psychosocial adversity [167] and combat [165], which accordingly could represent biomarkers of the brain related phenotype. In addition, substantial correlations between blood and brain samples have been observed in post-mortem studies [168]. On the other hand, the epigenetic modifications could be the result of PTSD effects on the HPA axis and immune system, as DNA methylation changes in response to environmental exposure can be induced by altered GC signalling [169].

There are also reports of intergenerational transmission of these epigenetic modifications [105,162], which could constitute one of the many mechanisms for intergenerational transmission of PTSD [28].

In brief, PTSD has been consistently associated with lower levels of cortisol and GR hypersensitivity. Furthermore, a meta-analysis found associations between variability in the *NR3C1* and *FKBP5* genes and PTSD. Other SNPs in genes involved in HPA axis regulation have also been found to be associated with PTSD, such as the *CRHR1*. Epigenome studies have found evidence of associations between levels of methylation in several genes with a regulatory role in HPA axis functioning—mainly *NR3C1* and *FKBP5*—which can depend on the gene's SNPs and on the gene's location of methylation. These findings are consistent with previous evidence of lower cortisol levels and GR hypersensitivity in

PTSD. All this genetic makeup variability has been found to interact with environmental influences, consubstantiating a new paradigm of gene × trauma × epigenetic interactions [155].

4. PTSD Treatments Which Influence the HPA Axis

4.1. GC Treatments

PTSD treatments using GR as a mediator have been tested for use as secondary prevention, that is to say, on exposure to a TE [54]. Based on studies which show that low peritraumatic cortisol constitutes a risk factor for PTSD development, GCs could be of benefit if administered immediately after the TE [170–173], especially in the case of individuals with this additional risk factor. A large randomised control study found that traumatic injury patients who received hydrocortisone within 12 h after trauma for 10 days reported fewer PTSD symptoms during the first three months post trauma than did patients who received a placebo [174]. On the other hand, GC antagonists could also be useful, based on the role of GCs in the consolidation of the traumatic memories [42]. As GC actions influence so many functions in the brain [46], the development of synthetic GCs or other GC action modulators with increased tissue/cell/molecular pathway selectivity could be of great benefit for patients, as they would act on the specific PTSD HPA axis-related pathophysiological mechanism [54,112]. However, research is still far from finding such "chirurgical" treatments.

Several clinical trials are currently being carried out with substances which aim to influence the HPA axis in PTSD patients [112]. These trials are supported by studies such as that by Aerni et al. [175]—a pilot study which found that a low dose of hydrocortisone administered over three months reduce re-experiencing and avoidance symptoms in PTSD patients, based on the assumption that elevated cortisol levels which inhibit memory retrieval in healthy human subjects can also reduce the excessive retrieval of traumatic memories and related symptoms in patients with chronic PTSD. Unfortunately, other larger placebo-controlled randomised trials targeting several HPA axis-related PTSD pathophysiological mechanisms did not achieve the same promising results [176–178].

Furthermore, hydrocortisone supplementation of prolonged exposure therapy for PTSD in military veterans has been associated with a lower dropout rate and greater reduction in total PTSD symptoms, when compared to a placebo [179]. Responders to hydrocortisone supplementation had the highest pre-treatment GC sensitivity, which decreased as symptoms improved.

Because *FKBP5* SNPs, methylation, and expression variation have all been consistently associated with PTSD pathophysiology, *FKBP5* is a potential treatment target, as it confers risk for abnormal fear extinction learning in humans [180].

A recent study by Pape et al. [181], which investigated the CRHR1 antagonist GSK561679 in female PTSD patients supports the possible role of *CRHR1* methylation levels as an epigenetic biomarker to follow response to CRHR1 antagonist treatment in specific subgroups. Moreover, pre-treatment *NR3C1* methylation levels may be useful as a potential biomarker to predict PTSD treatment outcome [33].

4.2. Psychotherapy for PTSD

Several psychotherapeutic interventions have been indicated for PTSD treatment. Some practice guidelines recommend them as first-line treatment [112,182,183]. Psychotherapeutic interventions for PTSD include both trauma-focussed ones, which are based on processing the emotional and cognitive aspects of the traumatic event, and non-trauma-focussed ones. Trauma-focussed approaches include prolonged exposure therapy (PE), cognitive processing therapy (CPT), and eye movement desensitisation and reprocessing (EMDR), which have all been considered first line psychotherapies [29,112]. On the other hand, stress inoculation training has been considered as first line non-trauma-focused psychotherapy for PTSD patients [29]. Recently, the guidelines are being increasingly questioned, as PE and CPT have high dropout rates, and only a minority of patients cease to be diagnosed with PTSD at the end of treatment [30,31]. Furthermore, recent trials have found no differences between several therapies, including the administration of sertraline hydrochloride and non-trauma-focussed therapies which were not previously considered to constitute first line psychotherapies for PTSD patients [31]. This highlights the importance of understanding the complexity and diversity of PTSD in each patient and also the need for the clinician to be able to adapt to the patient's needs, which can change over time [30]. Interestingly, Steenkamp et al. [31] state the need for long-term personalised approaches which can rely on the building of a therapeutic relationship to achieve better outcomes. Psychodynamic psychotherapies are also useful for the treatment of PTSD [184] and quality-based reviews of randomised controlled trials have shown no significant difference when compared with other psychotherapies, such as cognitive-behavioural therapy [185,186].

Psychotherapeutic interventions differ in a number of characteristics, such as the theoretical foundations, objectives, frequency of sessions, duration, required training of therapists, and the personal conditions required of potential candidates [187]. Although 30% of the results of psychotherapy are attributed to factors which are common to all of them [188], ideally we should use which ever psychotherapeutic intervention better works for each patient [189].

Daskalakis et al. [190] proposed a tree-hit model of the individual's programming sensitivity to environmental stress, depending on the timing of environmental exposure—should this have occurred during highly plastic developmental phases [191]. The genetic makeup (hit-1) interacts with early-life environmental exposure (hit-2), resulting in (endo) phenotypes (e.g., epigenetic changes and altered HPA axis function) [14] which constitute vulnerability or resilience factors, depending on the type and characteristics of later-life environmental challenges (hit-3) which confront the individual [190]. These later-life environmental challenges can also constitute the basis for psychotherapeutic repair when this three-hit model results in vulnerability and psychic suffering.

4.2.1. Psychotherapy and HPA Axis

PTSD is considered to be a memory-related fear disorder, which is characterised by an over-consolidation of TE-related fear, or, on the other hand, a failure to extinguish fear memories [54]. GCs have potentiating effects on emotional memories consolidation and impair memory retrieval. Several theories exist as to which mechanisms are involved in PTSD memory-related pathophysiology [54], including over-consolidation due to excessive noradrenergic signalling as a consequence of low levels of GCs [192] or due to GC-enhanced (as a result of GR hypersensitivity) fear memory consolidation [42]. After consolidation, memories can be retrieved. Important consequences after retrieval are the reconsolidation and extinction of memories, which seem to share the same role of GCs in both the amygdala and hippocampus as that of consolidation [54,193]. This is an important factor, as some PTSD psychotherapeutic interventions rely on fear learning paradigms which can be enhanced by GCs, depending on the knowledge of the adequate moment, dose, and choice of the GC to be administered. On the other hand, a GR antagonist might be more adequate if our aim is the GR hypersensitivity pathophysiological hypothesis of PTSD [54]. One example of this is the case of the most studied psychotherapy indicated for treatment of PTSD, that of PE, which relies on fear learning paradigms, particularly extinction learning, which, in turn, depend largely on the actions of GCs [54]. Extinction includes repeated presentations of the feared stimulus without reinforcement. Interindividual variability in extinction learning can be mediated in part by SNPs in *FKBP5* [180] and constitute one of the reasons for different treatment responses in patients with PTSD.

The first study to address the association of HPA axis-related risk factors with psychotherapeutic outcomes in PTSD patients showed that after brief eclectic psychotherapy, significant changes occurred in levels of cortisol and dehydroepiandrosterone in PTSD patients with civilian-related trauma. Those who responded to therapy showed an increase in cortisol and dehydroepiandrosterone levels, while for those who did not respond, both hormone levels decreased [32].

Accordingly, a higher bedtime salivary cortisol and 24-h urinary cortisol excretion predicted positive treatment outcomes in PTSD veterans after PE therapy or a weekly minimal attention intervention for 12 consecutive weeks [35]. Another study of combat-exposed male PTSD patients found that a high cortisol awakening response (CAR_i) before trauma-focussed psychotherapy predicted symptom reduction after 6–8 months. In this study, no differences were found between the PTSD and the non-PTSD group who had received no treatment with regard to a decrease in CAR_i at the end of the treatment period [194]. Furthermore, a study of veterans with PTSD showed that an increased salivary cortisol response to personal trauma script-driven imagery task prior to PTSD therapy was significantly and uniquely related to reductions in the core symptoms of PTSD after PE [195]. Interestingly, an 8-week psychosocial intervention with war-affected adolescents regulated hair cortisol levels. While this intervention decreased hair cortisol levels for young patients with hypersecretion and medium secretion, it increased hair cortisol levels for young patients with hyposecretion, in relation to the control group [196]. Steudte-Schmiedgen et al. [197] suggest that hair cortisol levels can be valuable to complement research into long-term HPA axis predictors and correlates of clinical outcomes in response to psychotherapy for PTSD patients.

A literature review revealed preliminary evidence that the lower levels of pre-treatment GC are related to poorer PTSD psychotherapeutic treatment gains [12]. The authors hypothesised that HPA axis dysregulation increases both behavioural and emotional avoidance, which interferes with the efficacy of psychotherapy, especially exposure-based interventions. This could constitute a strong argument for GC-enhanced psychotherapy. Another argument could be related to the fact that GCs can potentiate extinction learning [180] or decrease the retrieval of TEs memories on exposure to stimuli [198], either spontaneously [199], or during the application of PE therapy [179].

Imaging studies have also been carried out to understand whether structural modifications occur after psychotherapy. A metanalysis revealed that psychotherapy effects in PTSD increased prefrontal and decreased limbic activity, particularly by normalising hippocampal function and morphology [200]. Later studies continued to confirm these findings. Butler et al. [201] found hippocampal grey matter increases after six weeks of multimodal psychological treatment for combat-related PTSD, when compared with a waiting-list control group. Another study also found that clinical improvement during cognitive behavioural therapy in PTSD was predicted by increased *FKBP5* expression and increased hippocampal size [138]. Increased hippocampal volume and elevated *FKBP5* expression were significantly correlated. The hippocampus has been shown to be highly sensitive to the effects of GCs [202]. These studies highlight the key role that hippocampal neuroplasticity can play in improving resilience and recovery from traumatic stress, especially bearing in mind its involvement in the HPA axis regulation of memory extinction [54] and also that it is one of the major structures of neurogenesis in the adult human brain [203].

4.2.2. Psychotherapy Interaction with Genetic Makeup in PTSD

Since G × E interactions are determined by a certain confluence of environmental factors on SNPs and epigenomic mechanisms, and as these interactions exert an influence on the HPA axis-related pathophysiology of PTSD development and maintenance, we can accordingly presume that G × E interactions could be beneficial for the treatment of these and other disorders—if we could determine the terms of the interaction. In other words, what environmental change would be required for which genetic makeup? This environmental change could be a psychotherapeutic intervention.

Psychotherapeutic effects result from learning and memory-related neuronal plasticity [204] which ultimately depend on intervention-associated gene expression [205]). As SNPs and epigenetic changes have direct effects on gene expression, several lines of investigation have tried to better understand these relationships.

HPA axis-related genetic makeup information can be useful in psychotherapy practice through several of the following ways. Firstly, the SNPs of genes regulating the HPA axis function, such as *NR3C1*, *FKBP5*, and *CRHR1*, can interact with psychotherapeutic interventions in patients with specific PTSD characteristics and result in better outcomes. This knowledge can enable informed choices of the best intervention. Likewise, knowledge of the epigenome that is associated with better outcomes can also inform the decision regarding the most appropriate psychotherapy. This information could be constituted by biomarkers for both the indication and outcome of the psychotherapies for specific patients, as, for example, appears to happen in the case of a high level of pre-treatment cortisol as a predictor of better treatment outcomes [35,194,195]. In addition, psychotherapy addresses the trauma which seems to be the main culprit in HPA axis dysregulation interacting with genes.

Furthermore, the usefulness of genetic makeup information for the prescription of psychotherapy and the respective outcomes is promising, based on the results of several studies which have researched the interaction between psychotherapy and both SNPs and the epigenome.

The BclI SNP G carrier states predicted treatment gains after 12 consecutive weeks with PE therapy, or a weekly minimal attention intervention for patients with PTSD [35]. Homozygotes of the same BclI SNP risk allele evidenced more traumatic memories of intensive care unit treatment at six months after cardiac surgery [143]. Taken together, this information could help to identify those subjects who are at higher risk of PTSD symptoms and provide them with a psychotherapeutic intervention before, or shortly after the TE exposure, depending on its predictability. Interestingly, a randomised controlled trial study showed that a pre-operation minimal cognitive behavioural intervention which targeted homozygous carriers of this SNP's G high-risk allele reduced traumatic memories and posttraumatic stress disorder symptoms after heart surgery [206]. Interestingly, GG carriers of this SNP showed increased emotional memory performance when compared to GC and CC carriers [82].

Traumatised Ugandan carriers of the FKBP5 rs1360780 risk allele were at increased risk of PTSD symptoms relapse after 10 months of Narrative Exposure Therapy (a form of exposure-based short-term therapy), whereas non-carriers continued to show a reduction in symptoms [36]. This is an interesting result, as the genetic makeup which correlates with functional distinct roles impacts on different treatment outcomes [14,152].

Gene expression studies have also shown that increased FKBP5 expression after treatment is associated with successful response to trauma-focussed psychotherapy [33,138]. Levy-Gigi et al. [138] found significant increases in FKBP5 expression and in hippocampal size, which were correlated, in PTSD patients after 12 weekly 1.5-h sessions of trauma-focussed cognitive behavioural therapy. Improvement in PTSD symptoms was predicted by increased FKBP5 expression and increased hippocampal volume, although the primary predictor was FKBP5 expression [138].

A recent review of studies addressing the associations between various psychiatric disorders and several genes methylation before and after psychotherapeutic interventions concluded that DNA methylation change can be considered a marker of treatment outcome [100]. However, the author advises adopting caution in relation to the interpretation of results, owing to different methodologies across studies and also the need for the biological functional characterisation of the findings.

Higher NR3C1 exon 1_F promoter methylation levels predict a better treatment response after 12 weeks of PE psychotherapy, whereas FKBP5 exon 1 promoter region methylation levels decreased in those subjects who responded with remission to the same psychotherapy. Correspondingly, those subjects who responded to treatment had higher FKPP5 gene expression than those who did not respond [33]. The authors argue that GR gene methylation did not change in response to treatment, due to association with early environmental changes which could be more enduring. The methylation changes could constitute biomarkers of PTSD prognosis and symptom severity, respectively, as the environment part of G × E interactions could be attributed to epigenetic mechanisms [14].

Other studies addressing epigenomic mechanism in other genes associated with PTSD psychotherapy are currently being carried out. A longitudinal study of genome-wide DNA methylation levels found that the successful treatment of PTSD patients with trauma-focused psychotherapy (cognitive behavioural therapy, with or without EMDR) was accompanied by changes in DNA methylation at 12 differentially methylated genomic regions and particularly of the ZFP57 gene with regards to prospective evidence [34,207]. ZFP57 codes for a transcriptional regulator of genomic imprinting which has been associated with hippocampus-related stress vulnerability [208].

The previous research reviewed shows that the HPA axis is an important mediator of treatment approaches to PTSD, based on the fear learning paradigm of PTSD pathophysiology. Although promising, pharmacotherapy targeting the HPA axis still has a long way to go. In addition, GC-enhanced psychotherapy also represents a possible approach which needs to be investigated better. Indeed, psychotherapy research for treating PTSD needs to be pursued, as outcomes are far from good. It seems that certain endophenotypes can be useful in predicting treatment outcomes and psychotherapy has shown to normalise HPA axis-related functions in several ways, including levels or cortisol, gene expression, and CNS function and structure. The way genetic makeup (namely SNPs and DNA methylation) interacts with psychotherapy can also be useful to inform us of the best treatment options. However, further studies of these relationships are needed before we can apply these interesting discoveries to clinical practice.

5. Conclusions

5.1. Clinical Implications

PTSD is associated with many vulnerability and risk factors [6]. Several pathophysiological mechanisms have been hypothesised [54], which make this disorder phenotypically so diverse [19], and thus, treatments must inevitably be tailored, as we are now considering this disorder to be a gene–trauma–epigenetic interactions paradigm (Figure 3) [155].

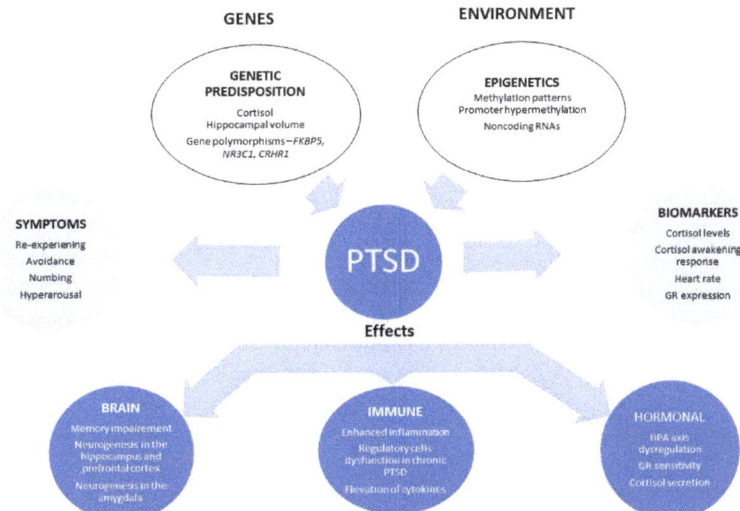

Figure 3. Gene/environment interaction in PTSD. Ranging from genetic and environment interactions through to symptoms, possible biomarkers and brain and hormonal changes. Abbreviations: HPA axis: hypothalamic–pituitary–adrenal axis; GR: glucocorticoid receptor. Adapted from [209].

Evidence is mounting that the HPA axis is implicated in PTSD pathophysiology and that interventions aiming to affect this system are showing increased usefulness for treatment interventions and can inform treatment outcomes—particularly psychotherapeutic interventions [e.g., 33,138,194].

We hope to have made it clear that traumatic experiences interact with the genetic makeup in several ways during human development. One of these is through modifications of the epigenome conditioning of the pathophysiology of many disorders—including PTSD. However, probably the most important message is that this interaction can occur reversely, through psychotherapeutic interventions which, if tailored according to the pathophysiological mechanisms, could be more useful for those individuals who suffer, and more cost-effective for all [33], although further studies need to be carried out to inform us better what works best, and for whom. If we could predict which patients would improve better with which type of treatment, then the level of suffering, time, and resources could be significantly reduced for such a complex and heterogeneous disorder. However, as promising and appealing the results of the studies reviewed in this paper might be, there is still a long way before they attain clinical applicability.

Furthermore, psychotherapy delivered perinatally with modifications which are specific to the perinatal period and are focussed on parenting are necessary for the prevention of PTSD intergenerational transmission [210], as PTSD influenced parent-child interactions are important and potentially modifiable contributors [211]. Evidence-based psychotherapy offers considerable advantages for perinatal PTSD, based on the potential teratogenic effects of typically-recommended medications for PTSD [212]. Furthermore, epigenetic modifications associated with PTSD are subject to inheritance [105]. If these epigenetic modifications could be reversed by psychotherapy, this would then constitute another way to break the intergenerational transmission of PTSD.

The studies mentioned in this review used psychotherapy for PTSD secondary or tertiary prevention or treatment, however, as it is known that there is a genetic risk for exposure to TEs, a primary psychotherapeutic intervention might also be useful, mainly for those individuals with other cumulative risk factors, such as childhood adversity or parental psychiatric disorders [6]. Furthermore, this review can also be useful to support the importance of trauma-informed care as a patient-centred approach which is needed in clinical practice and which can prevent many forms of trauma-related suffering [213].

5.2. Future Directions

Psychiatric disorders are multi-determined and have a complex pathophysiology and multiple phenotypic expressions, and therefore any information which could help tailor treatments should be pursued—in particular longitudinal gene × psychotherapy interaction studies.

In the case of PTSD, most of the psychotherapeutic interventions that have been studied are short-term, limited interventions. It would be interesting to study the effects of intensive interventions, which require treatments of more than once a week, with no time limits (e.g., psychoanalysis—which implies 3–5 sessions a week, also with no time limit). These interventions would address not only Daskalakis et al.'s [190] hit-3 environmental challenges, but also hit-2 early-life environmental exposure. What would be the changes in HPA axis biomarkers (endophenotypes) and the epigenetic changes? Would an association or interaction with SNPs of genes regulating HPA axis be found? Further research regarding the interactions between psychotherapy and the epigenome are warranted.

Studies are needed which focus on genetic makeup and their functional correlates, which can identify endophenotypes that constitute relevant mediators or moderators of treatment efficacy. A limited number of studies examine mRNA expression in relation to epigenetic modifications in patients with PTSD. This research is important, in order to find functional correlates between methylation patterns and phenotypic variability [71]. A better selection of the region to study DNA methylation also needs to be pursued, as well as other epigenetic mechanisms and their functional correlates [71,110]. In addition, larger samples should be studied to increase the study's power with randomised control trial approaches. Genome-wide studies of therapy responses would be ideal.

In the future, it should be possible to integrate different biomarkers—including SNPs, the epigenome, and gene expression profiles—with clinical variability and psychotherapeutic armamentarium with the objective to better inform those clinicians who practice personalised/patient-centred care for this complex and challenging disorder of PTSD.

Author Contributions: Conceptualisation, I.C.-V.; supervision, D.C.; methodology, I.C.-V.; visualisation, I.C.-V.; writing—original draft preparation, I.C.-V.; writing—review and editing, I.C.-V. and D.C. All authors have read and agreed to the published version of the manuscript.

Funding: This work was partially supported by the Associação dos Amigos do Serviço de Endocrinologia do Hospital de São João.

Conflicts of Interest: None of the authors have any conflict of interest to disclose.

References

1. American Psychiatric Association. *Diagnostic and Statistical Manual of Mental Disorders*, 5th ed.; American Psychiatric Association: Arlington, VA, USA, 2013.
2. Breslau, N.; Kessler, R.C.; Chilcoat, H.D.; Schultz, L.R.; Davis, G.C.; Andreski, P. Trauma and posttraumatic stress disorder in the community: The 1996 Detroit Area Survey of Trauma. *Arch. Gen. Psychiatry* **1998**, *55*, 626–632. [CrossRef] [PubMed]
3. Creamer, M.; Burgess, P.; McFarlane, A.C. Post-traumatic stress disorder: Findings from the Australian National Survey of Mental Health and Well-being. *Psychol. Med.* **2001**, *31*, 1237–1247. [CrossRef] [PubMed]
4. de Vries, G.J.; Olff, M. The lifetime prevalence of traumatic events and posttraumatic stress disorder in the Netherlands. *J. Trauma. Stress* **2009**, *22*, 259–267. [CrossRef] [PubMed]
5. Naifeh, J.A.; North, T.C.; Davis, J.L.; Reyes, G.; Logan, C.A.; Elhai, J.D. Clinical profile differences between PTSD-diagnosed military veterans and crime victims. *J. Trauma Dissociation Off. J. Int. Soc. Study Dissociation* **2008**, *9*, 321–334. [CrossRef] [PubMed]
6. Xue, C.; Ge, Y.; Tang, B.; Liu, Y.; Kang, P.; Wang, M.; Zhang, L. A meta-analysis of risk factors for combat-related PTSD among military personnel and veterans. *PLoS ONE* **2015**, *10*, e0120270. [CrossRef] [PubMed]
7. Herman, J.P.; McKlveen, J.M.; Ghosal, S.; Kopp, B.; Wulsin, A.; Makinson, R.; Scheimann, J.; Myers, B. Regulation of the Hypothalamic-Pituitary-Adrenocortical Stress Response. *Compr. Physiol.* **2016**, *6*, 603–621. [CrossRef]
8. Ramo-Fernandez, L.; Boeck, C.; Koenig, A.M.; Schury, K.; Binder, E.B.; Gundel, H.; Fegert, J.M.; Karabatsiakis, A.; Kolassa, I.T. The effects of childhood maltreatment on epigenetic regulation of stress-response associated genes: An intergenerational approach. *Sci. Rep.* **2019**, *9*, 983. [CrossRef]
9. Khoury, J.E.; Bosquet Enlow, M.; Plamondon, A.; Lyons-Ruth, K. The association between adversity and hair cortisol levels in humans: A meta-analysis. *Psychoneuroendocrinology* **2019**, *103*, 104–117. [CrossRef]
10. Castro-Vale, I.; van Rossum, E.F.; Machado, J.C.; Mota-Cardoso, R.; Carvalho, D. Genetics of glucocorticoid regulation and posttraumatic stress disorder–What do we know? *Neurosci. Biobehav. Rev.* **2016**, *63*, 143–157. [CrossRef]
11. Hawn, S.E.; Sheerin, C.M.; Lind, M.J.; Hicks, T.A.; Marraccini, M.E.; Bountress, K.; Bacanu, S.A.; Nugent, N.R.; Amstadter, A.B. GxE effects of FKBP5 and traumatic life events on PTSD: A meta-analysis. *J. Affect. Disord.* **2019**, *243*, 455–462. [CrossRef]
12. Colvonen, P.J.; Glassman, L.H.; Crocker, L.D.; Buttner, M.M.; Orff, H.; Schiehser, D.M.; Norman, S.B.; Afari, N. Pretreatment biomarkers predicting PTSD psychotherapy outcomes: A systematic review. *Neurosci. Biobehav. Rev.* **2017**, *75*, 140–156. [CrossRef] [PubMed]
13. Fernandez, C.A.; Choi, K.W.; Marshall, B.D.L.; Vicente, B.; Saldivia, S.; Kohn, R.; Koenen, K.C.; Arheart, K.L.; Buka, S.L. Assessing the relationship between psychosocial stressors and psychiatric resilience among Chilean disaster survivors. *Br. J. Psychiatry* **2020**, 1–8. [CrossRef] [PubMed]
14. Klengel, T.; Mehta, D.; Anacker, C.; Rex-Haffner, M.; Pruessner, J.C.; Pariante, C.M.; Pace, T.W.; Mercer, K.B.; Mayberg, H.S.; Bradley, B.; et al. Allele-specific FKBP5 DNA demethylation mediates gene-childhood trauma interactions. *Nat. Neurosci.* **2013**, *16*, 33–41. [CrossRef] [PubMed]
15. Mehta, D.; Miller, O.; Bruenig, D.; David, G.; Shakespeare-Finch, J. A Systematic Review of DNA Methylation and Gene Expression Studies in Posttraumatic Stress Disorder, Posttraumatic Growth, and Resilience. *J. Trauma Stress* **2020**, *33*, 171–180. [CrossRef]
16. Sartor, C.E.; Grant, J.D.; Lynskey, M.T.; McCutcheon, V.V.; Waldron, M.; Statham, D.J.; Bucholz, K.K.; Madden, P.A.; Heath, A.C.; Martin, N.G.; et al. Common heritable contributions to low-risk trauma, high-risk trauma, posttraumatic stress disorder, and major depression. *Arch. Gen. Psychiatry* **2012**, *69*, 293–299. [CrossRef] [PubMed]
17. True, W.R.; Rice, J.; Eisen, S.A.; Heath, A.C.; Goldberg, J.; Lyons, M.J.; Nowak, J. A twin study of genetic and environmental contributions to liability for posttraumatic stress symptoms. *Arch. Gen. Psychiatry* **1993**, *50*, 257–264. [CrossRef]
18. Sheerin, C.M.; Lind, M.J.; Bountress, K.E.; Marraccini, M.E.; Amstadter, A.B.; Bacanu, S.A.; Nugent, N.R. Meta-analysis of Associations Between Hypothalamic-Pituitary-Adrenal Axis Genes and Risk of Posttraumatic Stress Disorder. *J. Trauma Stress* **2020**. [CrossRef]

19. Galatzer-Levy, I.R.; Bryant, R.A. 636,120 Ways to Have Posttraumatic Stress Disorder. *Perspect. Psychol. Sci.* **2013**, *8*, 651–662. [CrossRef]
20. Bonanno, G.A.; Mancini, A.D.; Horton, J.L.; Powell, T.M.; Leardmann, C.A.; Boyko, E.J.; Wells, T.S.; Hooper, T.I.; Gackstetter, G.D.; Smith, T.C.; et al. Trajectories of trauma symptoms and resilience in deployed U.S. military service members: Prospective cohort study. *Br. J. Psychiatry* **2012**, *200*, 317–323. [CrossRef]
21. Bryant, R.A.; Nickerson, A.; Creamer, M.; O'Donnell, M.; Forbes, D.; Galatzer-Levy, I.; McFarlane, A.C.; Silove, D. Trajectory of post-traumatic stress following traumatic injury: 6-year follow-up. *Br. J. Psychiatry* **2015**, *206*, 417–423. [CrossRef]
22. Galatzer-Levy, I.R.; Madan, A.; Neylan, T.C.; Henn-Haase, C.; Marmar, C.R. Peritraumatic and trait dissociation differentiate police officers with resilient versus symptomatic trajectories of posttraumatic stress symptoms. *J. Trauma Stress* **2011**, *24*, 557–565. [CrossRef] [PubMed]
23. Pietrzak, R.H.; Van Ness, P.H.; Fried, T.R.; Galea, S.; Norris, F.H. Trajectories of posttraumatic stress symptomatology in older persons affected by a large-magnitude disaster. *J. Psychiatr. Res.* **2013**, *47*, 520–526. [CrossRef] [PubMed]
24. Kehle, S.M.; Reddy, M.K.; Ferrier-Auerbach, A.G.; Erbes, C.R.; Arbisi, P.A.; Polusny, M.A. Psychiatric diagnoses, comorbidity, and functioning in National Guard troops deployed to Iraq. *J. Psychiatr. Res.* **2011**, *45*, 126–132. [CrossRef] [PubMed]
25. Mellon, S.H.; Gautam, A.; Hammamieh, R.; Jett, M.; Wolkowitz, O.M. Metabolism, Metabolomics, and Inflammation in Posttraumatic Stress Disorder. *Biol. Psychiatry* **2018**, *83*, 866–875. [CrossRef]
26. Al-Turkait, F.A.; Ohaeri, J.U. Psychopathological status, behavior problems, and family adjustment of Kuwaiti children whose fathers were involved in the first gulf war. *Child. Adolesc. Psychiatry Ment. Health* **2008**, *2*, 12. [CrossRef] [PubMed]
27. Castro-Vale, I.; Severo, M.; Carvalho, D. Lifetime PTSD is associated with impaired emotion recognition in veterans and their offspring. *Psychiatry Res.* **2020**, *284*, 112666. [CrossRef] [PubMed]
28. Leen-Feldner, E.W.; Feldner, M.T.; Knapp, A.; Bunaciu, L.; Blumenthal, H.; Amstadter, A.B. Offspring psychological and biological correlates of parental posttraumatic stress: Review of the literature and research agenda. *Clin. Psychol. Rev.* **2013**, *33*, 1106–1133. [CrossRef]
29. Steenkamp, M.M.; Litz, B.T.; Hoge, C.W.; Marmar, C.R. Psychotherapy for Military-Related PTSD: A Review of Randomized Clinical Trials. *JAMA* **2015**, *314*, 489–500. [CrossRef]
30. Dimaggio, G. To expose or not to expose? The integrative therapist and posttraumatic stress disorder. *J. Psychother. Integr.* **2019**, *29*, 1–5. [CrossRef]
31. Steenkamp, M.M.; Litz, B.T.; Marmar, C.R. First-line Psychotherapies for Military-Related PTSD. *JAMA* **2020**, *323*, 656–657. [CrossRef]
32. Olff, M.; de Vries, G.J.; Guzelcan, Y.; Assies, J.; Gersons, B.P. Changes in cortisol and DHEA plasma levels after psychotherapy for PTSD. *Psychoneuroendocrinology* **2007**, *32*, 619–626. [CrossRef] [PubMed]
33. Yehuda, R.; Daskalakis, N.P.; Desarnaud, F.; Makotkine, I.; Lehrner, A.L.; Koch, E.; Flory, J.D.; Buxbaum, J.D.; Meaney, M.J.; Bierer, L.M. Epigenetic Biomarkers as Predictors and Correlates of Symptom Improvement Following Psychotherapy in Combat Veterans with PTSD. *Front. Psychiatry* **2013**, *4*, 118. [CrossRef] [PubMed]
34. Vinkers, C.H.; Geuze, E.; van Rooij, S.J.H.; Kennis, M.; Schur, R.R.; Nispeling, D.M.; Smith, A.K.; Nievergelt, C.M.; Uddin, M.; Rutten, B.P.F.; et al. Successful treatment of post-traumatic stress disorder reverses DNA methylation marks. *Mol. Psychiatry* **2019**. [CrossRef] [PubMed]
35. Yehuda, R.; Pratchett, L.C.; Elmes, M.W.; Lehrner, A.; Daskalakis, N.P.; Koch, E.; Makotkine, I.; Flory, J.D.; Bierer, L.M. Glucocorticoid-related predictors and correlates of post-traumatic stress disorder treatment response in combat veterans. *Interface Focus* **2014**, *4*, 20140048. [CrossRef] [PubMed]
36. Wilker, S.; Pfeiffer, A.; Kolassa, S.; Elbert, T.; Lingenfelder, B.; Ovuga, E.; Papassotiropoulos, A.; de Quervain, D.; Kolassa, I.T. The role of FKBP5 genotype in moderating long-term effectiveness of exposure-based psychotherapy for posttraumatic stress disorder. *Transl. Psychiatry* **2014**, *4*, e403. [CrossRef]
37. Antoni, F.A. Hypothalamic control of adrenocorticotropin secretion: Advances since the discovery of 41-residue corticotropin-releasing factor. *Endocr. Rev.* **1986**, *7*, 351–378. [CrossRef]
38. Gu, Y.; Piper, W.T.; Branigan, L.A.; Vazey, E.M.; Aston-Jones, G.; Lin, L.; LeDoux, J.E.; Sears, R.M. A brainstem-central amygdala circuit underlies defensive responses to learned threats. *Mol. Psychiatry* **2020**, *25*, 640–654. [CrossRef]

39. Bush, D.E.; Caparosa, E.M.; Gekker, A.; Ledoux, J. Beta-adrenergic receptors in the lateral nucleus of the amygdala contribute to the acquisition but not the consolidation of auditory fear conditioning. *Front. Behav. Neurosci.* **2010**, *4*, 154. [CrossRef]
40. Schiff, H.C.; Johansen, J.P.; Hou, M.; Bush, D.E.; Smith, E.K.; Klein, J.E.; LeDoux, J.E.; Sears, R.M. beta-Adrenergic Receptors Regulate the Acquisition and Consolidation Phases of Aversive Memory Formation Through Distinct, Temporally Regulated Signaling Pathways. *Neuropsychopharmacology* **2017**, *42*, 895–903. [CrossRef]
41. Jedema, H.P.; Grace, A.A. Corticotropin-releasing hormone directly activates noradrenergic neurons of the locus ceruleus recorded in vitro. *J. Neurosci. Off. J. Soc. Neurosci.* **2004**, *24*, 9703–9713. [CrossRef]
42. de Quervain, D.; Schwabe, L.; Roozendaal, B. Stress, glucocorticoids and memory: Implications for treating fear-related disorders. *Nat. Rev. Neurosci.* **2017**, *18*, 7–19. [CrossRef] [PubMed]
43. Groeneweg, F.L.; Karst, H.; de Kloet, E.R.; Joels, M. Rapid non-genomic effects of corticosteroids and their role in the central stress response. *J. Endocrinol.* **2011**, *209*, 153–167. [CrossRef] [PubMed]
44. Pape, H.C.; Pare, D. Plastic synaptic networks of the amygdala for the acquisition, expression, and extinction of conditioned fear. *Physiol. Rev.* **2010**, *90*, 419–463. [CrossRef] [PubMed]
45. Lightman, S.L.; Wiles, C.C.; Atkinson, H.C.; Henley, D.E.; Russell, G.M.; Leendertz, J.A.; McKenna, M.A.; Spiga, F.; Wood, S.A.; Conway-Campbell, B.L. The significance of glucocorticoid pulsatility. *Eur J. Pharm.* **2008**, *583*, 255–262. [CrossRef]
46. Juszczak, G.R.; Stankiewicz, A.M. Glucocorticoids, genes and brain function. *Prog. Neuropsychopharmacol. Biol. Psychiatry* **2018**, *82*, 136–168. [CrossRef]
47. Roozendaal, B.; McEwen, B.S.; Chattarji, S. Stress, memory and the amygdala. *Nat. Rev. Neurosci.* **2009**, *10*, 423–433. [CrossRef]
48. Papadimitriou, A.; Priftis, K.N. Regulation of the hypothalamic-pituitary-adrenal axis. *Neuroimmunomodulation* **2009**, *16*, 265–271. [CrossRef]
49. Moisan, M.P.; Minni, A.M.; Dominguez, G.; Helbling, J.C.; Foury, A.; Henkous, N.; Dorey, R.; Beracochea, D. Role of corticosteroid binding globulin in the fast actions of glucocorticoids on the brain. *Steroids* **2014**, *81*, 109–115. [CrossRef]
50. Wyrwoll, C.S.; Holmes, M.C.; Seckl, J.R. 11beta-hydroxysteroid dehydrogenases and the brain: From zero to hero, a decade of progress. *Front. Neuroendocr.* **2011**, *32*, 265–286. [CrossRef]
51. Quax, R.A.; Manenschijn, L.; Koper, J.W.; Hazes, J.M.; Lamberts, S.W.; van Rossum, E.F.; Feelders, R.A. Glucocorticoid sensitivity in health and disease. *Nat. Rev. Endocrinol.* **2013**, *9*, 670–686. [CrossRef] [PubMed]
52. Vamvakopoulos, N.V. Sexual dimorphism of stress response and immune/inflammatory reaction: The corticotropin releasing hormone perspective. *Mediat. Inflamm.* **1995**, *4*, 163–174. [CrossRef] [PubMed]
53. Weiss, E.L.; Longhurst, J.G.; Mazure, C.M. Childhood sexual abuse as a risk factor for depression in women: Psychosocial and neurobiological correlates. *Am. J. Psychiatry* **1999**, *156*, 816–828. [CrossRef] [PubMed]
54. Dunlop, B.W.; Wong, A. The hypothalamic-pituitary-adrenal axis in PTSD: Pathophysiology and treatment interventions. *Prog. Neuropsychopharmacol. Biol. Psychiatry* **2019**, *89*, 361–379. [CrossRef] [PubMed]
55. Reul, J.M.; de Kloet, E.R. Two receptor systems for corticosterone in rat brain: Microdistribution and differential occupation. *Endocrinology* **1985**, *117*, 2505–2511. [CrossRef]
56. de Kloet, E.R. From receptor balance to rational glucocorticoid therapy. *Endocrinology* **2014**, *155*, 2754–2769. [CrossRef] [PubMed]
57. Nishi, M.; Kawata, M. Dynamics of glucocorticoid receptor and mineralocorticoid receptor: Implications from live cell imaging studies. *Neuroendocrinology* **2007**, *85*, 186–192. [CrossRef]
58. Ramamoorthy, S.; Cidlowski, J.A. Corticosteroids: Mechanisms of Action in Health and Disease. *Rheum. Dis. Clin. N. Am.* **2016**, *42*, 15–31. [CrossRef]
59. Oakley, R.H.; Cidlowski, J.A. Cellular processing of the glucocorticoid receptor gene and protein: New mechanisms for generating tissue-specific actions of glucocorticoids. *J. Biol. Chem.* **2011**, *286*, 3177–3184. [CrossRef] [PubMed]
60. Oakley, R.H.; Cidlowski, J.A. The biology of the glucocorticoid receptor: New signaling mechanisms in health and disease. *J. Allergy Clin. Immunol.* **2013**, *132*, 1033–1044. [CrossRef] [PubMed]
61. Jiang, S.; Postovit, L.; Cattaneo, A.; Binder, E.B.; Aitchison, K.J. Epigenetic Modifications in Stress Response Genes Associated With Childhood Trauma. *Front. Psychiatry* **2019**, *10*, 808. [CrossRef] [PubMed]

62. Derijk, R.H.; Schaaf, M.J.; Turner, G.; Datson, N.A.; Vreugdenhil, E.; Cidlowski, J.; de Kloet, E.R.; Emery, P.; Sternberg, E.M.; Detera-Wadleigh, S.D. A human glucocorticoid receptor gene variant that increases the stability of the glucocorticoid receptor beta-isoform mRNA is associated with rheumatoid arthritis. *J. Rheumatol.* **2001**, *28*, 2383–2388. [PubMed]
63. Grad, I.; Picard, D. The glucocorticoid responses are shaped by molecular chaperones. *Mol. Cell Endocrinol.* **2007**, *275*, 2–12. [CrossRef] [PubMed]
64. Vandevyver, S.; Dejager, L.; Van Bogaert, T.; Kleyman, A.; Liu, Y.; Tuckermann, J.; Libert, C. Glucocorticoid receptor dimerization induces MKP1 to protect against TNF-induced inflammation. *J. Clin. Investig.* **2012**, *122*, 2130–2140. [CrossRef] [PubMed]
65. Groeneweg, F.L.; Karst, H.; de Kloet, E.R.; Joels, M. Mineralocorticoid and glucocorticoid receptors at the neuronal membrane, regulators of nongenomic corticosteroid signalling. *Mol. Cell Endocrinol.* **2012**, *350*, 299–309. [CrossRef] [PubMed]
66. Atsak, P.; Roozendaal, B.; Campolongo, P. Role of the endocannabinoid system in regulating glucocorticoid effects on memory for emotional experiences. *Neuroscience* **2012**, *204*, 104–116. [CrossRef]
67. Vernocchi, S.; Battello, N.; Schmitz, S.; Revets, D.; Billing, A.M.; Turner, J.D.; Muller, C.P. Membrane glucocorticoid receptor activation induces proteomic changes aligning with classical glucocorticoid effects. *Mol. Cell Proteom. MCP* **2013**, *12*, 1764–1779. [CrossRef]
68. Binder, E.B. The role of FKBP5, a co-chaperone of the glucocorticoid receptor in the pathogenesis and therapy of affective and anxiety disorders. *Psychoneuroendocrinology* **2009**, *34* (Suppl. 1), S186–S195. [CrossRef]
69. Vermeer, H.; Hendriks-Stegeman, B.I.; van der Burg, B.; van Buul-Offers, S.C.; Jansen, M. Glucocorticoid-induced increase in lymphocytic FKBP51 messenger ribonucleic acid expression: A potential marker for glucocorticoid sensitivity, potency, and bioavailability. *J. Clin. Endocrinol. Metab.* **2003**, *88*, 277–284. [CrossRef]
70. Evans, R.M. The steroid and thyroid hormone receptor superfamily. *Science (NY)* **1988**, *240*, 889–895. [CrossRef]
71. Palma-Gudiel, H.; Cordova-Palomera, A.; Leza, J.C.; Fananas, L. Glucocorticoid receptor gene (NR3C1) methylation processes as mediators of early adversity in stress-related disorders causality: A critical review. *Neurosci. Biobehav. Rev.* **2015**, *55*, 520–535. [CrossRef]
72. Cao-Lei, L.; Leija, S.C.; Kumsta, R.; Wust, S.; Meyer, J.; Turner, J.D.; Muller, C.P. Transcriptional control of the human glucocorticoid receptor: Identification and analysis of alternative promoter regions. *Hum. Genet.* **2011**, *129*, 533–543. [CrossRef] [PubMed]
73. Manenschijn, L.; van den Akker, E.L.; Lamberts, S.W.; van Rossum, E.F. Clinical features associated with glucocorticoid receptor polymorphisms. An overview. *Ann. NY Acad. Sci.* **2009**, *1179*, 179–198. [CrossRef] [PubMed]
74. van Rossum, E.F.; Roks, P.H.; de Jong, F.H.; Brinkmann, A.O.; Pols, H.A.; Koper, J.W.; Lamberts, S.W. Characterization of a promoter polymorphism in the glucocorticoid receptor gene and its relationship to three other polymorphisms. *Clin. Endocrinol. (Oxf.)* **2004**, *61*, 573–581. [CrossRef] [PubMed]
75. Koper, J.W.; Stolk, R.P.; de Lange, P.; Huizenga, N.A.; Molijn, G.J.; Pols, H.A.; Grobbee, D.E.; Karl, M.; de Jong, F.H.; Brinkmann, A.O.; et al. Lack of association between five polymorphisms in the human glucocorticoid receptor gene and glucocorticoid resistance. *Hum. Genet.* **1997**, *99*, 663–668. [CrossRef] [PubMed]
76. Russcher, H.; Smit, P.; van den Akker, E.L.; van Rossum, E.F.; Brinkmann, A.O.; de Jong, F.H.; Lamberts, S.W.; Koper, J.W. Two polymorphisms in the glucocorticoid receptor gene directly affect glucocorticoid-regulated gene expression. *J. Clin. Endocrinol. Metab.* **2005**, *90*, 5804–5810. [CrossRef]
77. van Rossum, E.F.; Koper, J.W.; Huizenga, N.A.; Uitterlinden, A.G.; Janssen, J.A.; Brinkmann, A.O.; Grobbee, D.E.; de Jong, F.H.; van Duyn, C.M.; Pols, H.A.; et al. A polymorphism in the glucocorticoid receptor gene, which decreases sensitivity to glucocorticoids in vivo, is associated with low insulin and cholesterol levels. *Diabetes* **2002**, *51*, 3128–3134. [CrossRef]
78. Russcher, H.; van Rossum, E.F.; de Jong, F.H.; Brinkmann, A.O.; Lamberts, S.W.; Koper, J.W. Increased expression of the glucocorticoid receptor-A translational isoform as a result of the ER22/23EK polymorphism. *Mol. Endocrinol.* **2005**, *19*, 1687–1696. [CrossRef]

79. Huizenga, N.A.; Koper, J.W.; De Lange, P.; Pols, H.A.; Stolk, R.P.; Burger, H.; Grobbee, D.E.; Brinkmann, A.O.; De Jong, F.H.; Lamberts, S.W. A polymorphism in the glucocorticoid receptor gene may be associated with and increased sensitivity to glucocorticoids in vivo. *J. Clin. Endocrinol. Metab.* **1998**, *83*, 144–151. [CrossRef]
80. van Rossum, E.F.; Koper, J.W.; van den Beld, A.W.; Uitterlinden, A.G.; Arp, P.; Ester, W.; Janssen, J.A.; Brinkmann, A.O.; de Jong, F.H.; Grobbee, D.E.; et al. Identification of the BclI polymorphism in the glucocorticoid receptor gene: Association with sensitivity to glucocorticoids in vivo and body mass index. *Clin. Endocrinol. (Oxf.)* **2003**, *59*, 585–592. [CrossRef]
81. Panarelli, M.; Holloway, C.D.; Fraser, R.; Connell, J.M.; Ingram, M.C.; Anderson, N.H.; Kenyon, C.J. Glucocorticoid receptor polymorphism, skin vasoconstriction, and other metabolic intermediate phenotypes in normal human subjects. *J. Clin. Endocrinol. Metab.* **1998**, *83*, 1846–1852. [CrossRef]
82. Ackermann, S.; Heck, A.; Rasch, B.; Papassotiropoulos, A.; de Quervain, D.J. The BclI polymorphism of the glucocorticoid receptor gene is associated with emotional memory performance in healthy individuals. *Psychoneuroendocrinology* **2013**, *38*, 1203–1207. [CrossRef] [PubMed]
83. Kumsta, R.; Entringer, S.; Koper, J.W.; van Rossum, E.F.; Hellhammer, D.H.; Wust, S. Sex specific associations between common glucocorticoid receptor gene variants and hypothalamus-pituitary-adrenal axis responses to psychosocial stress. *Biol. Psychiatry* **2007**, *62*, 863–869. [CrossRef] [PubMed]
84. van den Akker, E.L.; Russcher, H.; van Rossum, E.F.; Brinkmann, A.O.; de Jong, F.H.; Hokken, A.; Pols, H.A.; Koper, J.W.; Lamberts, S.W. Glucocorticoid receptor polymorphism affects transrepression but not transactivation. *J. Clin. Endocrinol. Metab.* **2006**, *91*, 2800–2803. [CrossRef] [PubMed]
85. Lian, Y.; Xiao, J.; Wang, Q.; Ning, L.; Guan, S.; Ge, H.; Li, F.; Liu, J. The relationship between glucocorticoid receptor polymorphisms, stressful life events, social support, and post-traumatic stress disorder. *BMC Psychiatry* **2014**, *14*, 232. [CrossRef]
86. Marceca, C.; Pfob, M.; Schelling, G.; Steinlein, O.K.; Eggert, M. Single nucleotide polymorphism creating a variable upstream open reading frame regulates glucocorticoid receptor expression. *Gene* **2015**, *563*, 24–28. [CrossRef]
87. Szczepankiewicz, A.; Leszczynska-Rodziewicz, A.; Pawlak, J.; Rajewska-Rager, A.; Dmitrzak-Weglarz, M.; Wilkosc, M.; Skibinska, M.; Hauser, J. Glucocorticoid receptor polymorphism is associated with major depression and predominance of depression in the course of bipolar disorder. *J. Affect. Disord.* **2011**, *134*, 138–144. [CrossRef] [PubMed]
88. van West, D.; Van Den Eede, F.; Del-Favero, J.; Souery, D.; Norrback, K.F.; Van Duijn, C.; Sluijs, S.; Adolfsson, R.; Mendlewicz, J.; Deboutte, D.; et al. Glucocorticoid receptor gene-based SNP analysis in patients with recurrent major depression. *Neuropsychopharmacology* **2006**, *31*, 620–627. [CrossRef]
89. Nair, S.C.; Rimerman, R.A.; Toran, E.J.; Chen, S.; Prapapanich, V.; Butts, R.N.; Smith, D.F. Molecular cloning of human FKBP51 and comparisons of immunophilin interactions with Hsp90 and progesterone receptor. *Mol. Cell Biol.* **1997**, *17*, 594–603. [CrossRef] [PubMed]
90. Reynolds, P.D.; Ruan, Y.; Smith, D.F.; Scammell, J.G. Glucocorticoid resistance in the squirrel monkey is associated with overexpression of the immunophilin FKBP51. *J. Clin. Endocrinol. Metab.* **1999**, *84*, 663–669. [CrossRef]
91. Zannas, A.S.; Wiechmann, T.; Gassen, N.C.; Binder, E.B. Gene-Stress-Epigenetic Regulation of FKBP5: Clinical and Translational Implications. *Neuropsychopharmacology* **2016**, *41*, 261–274. [CrossRef]
92. Binder, E.B.; Salyakina, D.; Lichtner, P.; Wochnik, G.M.; Ising, M.; Putz, B.; Papiol, S.; Seaman, S.; Lucae, S.; Kohli, M.A.; et al. Polymorphisms in FKBP5 are associated with increased recurrence of depressive episodes and rapid response to antidepressant treatment. *Nat. Genet.* **2004**, *36*, 1319–1325. [CrossRef] [PubMed]
93. Binder, E.B.; Bradley, R.G.; Liu, W.; Epstein, M.P.; Deveau, T.C.; Mercer, K.B.; Tang, Y.; Gillespie, C.F.; Heim, C.M.; Nemeroff, C.B.; et al. Association of FKBP5 polymorphisms and childhood abuse with risk of posttraumatic stress disorder symptoms in adults. *JAMA* **2008**, *299*, 1291–1305. [CrossRef] [PubMed]
94. Klengel, T.; Binder, E.B. FKBP5 allele-specific epigenetic modification in gene by environment interaction. *Neuropsychopharmacology* **2015**, *40*, 244–246. [CrossRef] [PubMed]
95. Amstadter, A.B.; Nugent, N.R.; Yang, B.Z.; Miller, A.; Siburian, R.; Moorjani, P.; Haddad, S.; Basu, A.; Fagerness, J.; Saxe, G.; et al. Corticotrophin-releasing hormone type 1 receptor gene (CRHR1) variants predict posttraumatic stress disorder onset and course in pediatric injury patients. *Dis. Mark.* **2011**, *30*, 89–99. [CrossRef]

96. White, S.; Acierno, R.; Ruggiero, K.J.; Koenen, K.C.; Kilpatrick, D.G.; Galea, S.; Gelernter, J.; Williamson, V.; McMichael, O.; Vladimirov, V.I.; et al. Association of CRHR1 variants and posttraumatic stress symptoms in hurricane exposed adults. *J. Anxiety Disord.* **2013**, *27*, 678–683. [CrossRef]
97. Halldorsdottir, T.; Binder, E.B. Gene x Environment Interactions: From Molecular Mechanisms to Behavior. *Annu. Rev. Psychol.* **2017**, *68*, 215–241. [CrossRef]
98. Heim, C.; Bradley, B.; Mletzko, T.C.; Deveau, T.C.; Musselman, D.L.; Nemeroff, C.B.; Ressler, K.J.; Binder, E.B. Effect of Childhood Trauma on Adult Depression and Neuroendocrine Function: Sex-Specific Moderation by CRH Receptor 1 Gene. *Front. Behav. Neurosci.* **2009**, *3*, 41. [CrossRef]
99. Webb, L.M.; Phillips, K.E.; Ho, M.C.; Veldic, M.; Blacker, C.J. The Relationship between DNA Methylation and Antidepressant Medications: A Systematic Review. *Int. J. Mol. Sci.* **2020**, *21*. [CrossRef]
100. Kumsta, R. The role of epigenetics for understanding mental health difficulties and its implications for psychotherapy research. *Psychol. Psychother.* **2019**, *92*, 190–207. [CrossRef]
101. Howie, H.; Rijal, C.M.; Ressler, K.J. A review of epigenetic contributions to post-traumatic stress disorder. *Dialogues Clin. Neurosci.* **2019**, *21*, 417–428. [CrossRef]
102. Daskalakis, N.P.; Rijal, C.M.; King, C.; Huckins, L.M.; Ressler, K.J. Recent Genetics and Epigenetics Approaches to PTSD. *Curr. Psychiatry Rep.* **2018**, *20*, 30. [CrossRef] [PubMed]
103. Sweatt, J.D.; Meaney, M.J.P.; Nestler, E.J.; Akbarian, S. *Epigenetic Regulation in the Nervous System: Basic Mechanisms and Clinical Impact*; Sweatt, J.D., Meaney, M.J.P., Nestler, E.J., Akbarian, S., Eds.; Academic Press: San Diego, CA, USA, 2013.
104. Wei, J.W.; Huang, K.; Yang, C.; Kang, C.S. Non-coding RNAs as regulators in epigenetics (Review). *Oncol. Rep.* **2017**, *37*, 3–9. [CrossRef] [PubMed]
105. Bohacek, J.; Mansuy, I.M. Molecular insights into transgenerational non-genetic inheritance of acquired behaviours. *Nat. Rev. Genet.* **2015**, *16*, 641–652. [CrossRef] [PubMed]
106. Dias, B.G.; Maddox, S.; Klengel, T.; Ressler, K.J. Epigenetic mechanisms underlying learning and the inheritance of learned behaviors. *Trends Neurosci.* **2015**, *38*, 96–107. [CrossRef] [PubMed]
107. Kappeler, L.; Meaney, M.J. Epigenetics and parental effects. *Bioessays* **2010**, *32*, 818–827. [CrossRef]
108. McGowan, P.O.; Sasaki, A.; D'Alessio, A.C.; Dymov, S.; Labonte, B.; Szyf, M.; Turecki, G.; Meaney, M.J. Epigenetic regulation of the glucocorticoid receptor in human brain associates with childhood abuse. *Nat. Neurosci.* **2009**, *12*, 342–348. [CrossRef]
109. Linnstaedt, S.D.; Riker, K.D.; Rueckeis, C.A.; Kutchko, K.M.; Lackey, L.; McCarthy, K.R.; Tsai, Y.H.; Parker, J.S.; Kurz, M.C.; Hendry, P.L.; et al. A Functional riboSNitch in the 3′ Untranslated Region of FKBP5 Alters MicroRNA-320a Binding Efficiency and Mediates Vulnerability to Chronic Post-Traumatic Pain. *J. Neurosci. Off. J. Soc. Neurosci.* **2018**, *38*, 8407–8420. [CrossRef]
110. Daskalakis, N.P.; Provost, A.C.; Hunter, R.G.; Guffanti, G. Noncoding RNAs: Stress, Glucocorticoids, and Posttraumatic Stress Disorder. *Biol. Psychiatry* **2018**, *83*, 849–865. [CrossRef]
111. Heim, C.; Nemeroff, C.B. Neurobiology of posttraumatic stress disorder. *CNS Spectr.* **2009**, *14*, 13–24.
112. Yehuda, R.; Hoge, C.W.; McFarlane, A.C.; Vermetten, E.; Lanius, R.A.; Nievergelt, C.M.; Hobfoll, S.E.; Koenen, K.C.; Neylan, T.C.; Hyman, S.E. Post-traumatic stress disorder. *Nat. Rev. Dis. Primers* **2015**, *1*, 15057. [CrossRef]
113. Daskalakis, N.P.; Lehrner, A.; Yehuda, R. Endocrine aspects of post-traumatic stress disorder and implications for diagnosis and treatment. *Endocrinol. Metab. Clin. N. Am.* **2013**, *42*, 503–513. [CrossRef] [PubMed]
114. Barker, E.D.; Walton, E.; Cecil, C.A.M. Annual Research Review: DNA methylation as a mediator in the association between risk exposure and child and adolescent psychopathology. *J. Child. Psychol. Psychiatryand Allied Discip.* **2018**, *59*, 303–322. [CrossRef] [PubMed]
115. Kornfield, S.L.; Hantsoo, L.; Epperson, C.N. What Does Sex Have to Do with It? The Role of Sex as a Biological Variable in the Development of Posttraumatic Stress Disorder. *Curr. Psychiatry Rep.* **2018**, *20*, 39. [CrossRef]
116. Olff, M.; Langeland, W.; Draijer, N.; Gersons, B.P. Gender differences in posttraumatic stress disorder. *Psychol. Bull.* **2007**, *33*, 183–204. [CrossRef] [PubMed]
117. Quide, Y.; Andersson, F.; Dufour-Rainfray, D.; Descriaud, C.; Brizard, B.; Gissot, V.; Clery, H.; Carrey Le Bas, M.P.; Osterreicher, S.; Ogielska, M.; et al. Smaller hippocampal volume following sexual assault in women is associated with post-traumatic stress disorder. *Acta Psychiatr. Scand.* **2018**, *138*, 312–324. [CrossRef] [PubMed]

118. Morris, M.C.; Compas, B.E.; Garber, J. Relations among posttraumatic stress disorder, comorbid major depression, and HPA function: A systematic review and meta-analysis. *Clin. Psychol. Rev.* **2012**, *32*, 301–315. [CrossRef]
119. Yehuda, R.; Golier, J.A.; Halligan, S.L.; Meaney, M.; Bierer, L.M. The ACTH response to dexamethasone in PTSD. *Am. J. Psychiatry* **2004**, *161*, 1397–1403. [CrossRef]
120. Yehuda, R.; Golier, J.A.; Yang, R.K.; Tischler, L. Enhanced sensitivity to glucocorticoids in peripheral mononuclear leukocytes in posttraumatic stress disorder. *Biol. Psychiatry* **2004**, *55*, 1110–1116. [CrossRef]
121. McFarlane, A.C.; Barton, C.A.; Yehuda, R.; Wittert, G. Cortisol response to acute trauma and risk of posttraumatic stress disorder. *Psychoneuroendocrinology* **2011**, *36*, 720–727. [CrossRef]
122. Rohleder, N.; Wolf, J.M.; Wolf, O.T. Glucocorticoid sensitivity of cognitive and inflammatory processes in depression and posttraumatic stress disorder. *Neurosci. Biobehav. Rev.* **2010**, *35*, 104–114. [CrossRef]
123. Meewisse, M.L.; Reitsma, J.B.; de Vries, G.J.; Gersons, B.P.; Olff, M. Cortisol and post-traumatic stress disorder in adults: Systematic review and meta-analysis. *Br. J. Psychiatry* **2007**, *191*, 387–392. [CrossRef] [PubMed]
124. Pan, X.; Wang, Z.; Wu, X.; Wen, S.W.; Liu, A. Salivary cortisol in post-traumatic stress disorder: A systematic review and meta-analysis. *BMC Psychiatry* **2018**, *18*, 324. [CrossRef] [PubMed]
125. Pan, X.; Kaminga, A.C.; Wen, S.W.; Wang, Z.; Wu, X.; Liu, A. The 24-hour urinary cortisol in post-traumatic stress disorder: A meta-analysis. *PLoS ONE* **2020**, *15*, e0227560. [CrossRef] [PubMed]
126. Wang, L.; Cao, C.; Wang, W.; Xu, H.; Zhang, J.; Deng, H.; Zhang, X. Linking hair cortisol levels to phenotypic heterogeneity of posttraumatic stress symptoms in highly traumatized chinese women. *Biol. Psychiatry* **2015**, *77*, e21–e22. [CrossRef] [PubMed]
127. Steudte, S.; Kirschbaum, C.; Gao, W.; Alexander, N.; Schonfeld, S.; Hoyer, J.; Stalder, T. Hair cortisol as a biomarker of traumatization in healthy individuals and posttraumatic stress disorder patients. *Biol. Psychiatry* **2013**, *74*, 639–646. [CrossRef]
128. Sautter, F.J.; Bissette, G.; Wiley, J.; Manguno-Mire, G.; Schoenbachler, B.; Myers, L.; Johnson, J.E.; Cerbone, A.; Malaspina, D. Corticotropin-releasing factor in posttraumatic stress disorder (PTSD) with secondary psychotic symptoms, nonpsychotic PTSD, and healthy control subjects. *Biol. Psychiatry* **2003**, *54*, 1382–1388. [CrossRef]
129. Baker, D.G.; West, S.A.; Nicholson, W.E.; Ekhator, N.N.; Kasckow, J.W.; Hill, K.K.; Bruce, A.B.; Orth, D.N.; Geracioti, T.D., Jr. Serial CSF corticotropin-releasing hormone levels and adrenocortical activity in combat veterans with posttraumatic stress disorder. *Am. J. Psychiatry* **1999**, *156*, 585–588. [CrossRef] [PubMed]
130. Bremner, J.D.; Licinio, J.; Darnell, A.; Krystal, J.H.; Owens, M.J.; Southwick, S.M.; Nemeroff, C.B.; Charney, D.S. Elevated CSF corticotropin-releasing factor concentrations in posttraumatic stress disorder. *Am. J. Psychiatry* **1997**, *154*, 624–629. [CrossRef]
131. Raison, C.L.; Miller, A.H. When not enough is too much: The role of insufficient glucocorticoid signaling in the pathophysiology of stress-related disorders. *Am. J. Psychiatry* **2003**, *160*, 1554–1565. [CrossRef]
132. Mahan, A.L.; Ressler, K.J. Fear conditioning, synaptic plasticity and the amygdala: Implications for posttraumatic stress disorder. *Trends Neurosci.* **2012**, *35*, 24–35. [CrossRef]
133. van Zuiden, M.; Geuze, E.; Willemen, H.L.; Vermetten, E.; Maas, M.; Amarouchi, K.; Kavelaars, A.; Heijnen, C.J. Glucocorticoid receptor pathway components predict posttraumatic stress disorder symptom development: A prospective study. *Biol. Psychiatry* **2012**, *71*, 309–316. [CrossRef] [PubMed]
134. Galatzer-Levy, I.R.; Steenkamp, M.M.; Brown, A.D.; Qian, M.; Inslisht, S.; Henn-Haase, C.; Otte, C.; Yehuda, R.; Neylan, T.C.; Marmar, C.R. Cortisol response to an experimental stress paradigm prospectively predicts long-term distress and resilience trajectories in response to active police service. *J. Psychiatr. Res.* **2014**, *56*, 36–42. [CrossRef] [PubMed]
135. Steudte-Schmiedgen, S.; Stalder, T.; Schonfeld, S.; Wittchen, H.U.; Trautmann, S.; Alexander, N.; Miller, R.; Kirschbaum, C. Hair cortisol concentrations and cortisol stress reactivity predict PTSD symptom increase after trauma exposure during military deployment. *Psychoneuroendocrinology* **2015**, *59*, 123–133. [CrossRef] [PubMed]
136. Resnick, H.S.; Yehuda, R.; Pitman, R.K.; Foy, D.W. Effect of previous trauma on acute plasma cortisol level following rape. *Am. J. Psychiatry* **1995**, *152*, 1675–1677. [CrossRef]
137. Morris, M.C.; Hellman, N.; Abelson, J.L.; Rao, U. Cortisol, heart rate, and blood pressure as early markers of PTSD risk: A systematic review and meta-analysis. *Clin. Psychol. Rev.* **2016**, *49*, 79–91. [CrossRef]

138. Levy-Gigi, E.; Szabo, C.; Kelemen, O.; Keri, S. Association among clinical response, hippocampal volume, and FKBP5 gene expression in individuals with posttraumatic stress disorder receiving cognitive behavioral therapy. *Biol. Psychiatry* **2013**, *74*, 793–800. [CrossRef]
139. Childress, J.E.; McDowell, E.J.; Dalai, V.V.; Bogale, S.R.; Ramamurthy, C.; Jawaid, A.; Kunik, M.E.; Qureshi, S.U.; Schulz, P.E. Hippocampal volumes in patients with chronic combat-related posttraumatic stress disorder: A systematic review. *J. Neuropsychiatry Clin. Neurosci* **2013**, *25*, 12–25. [CrossRef]
140. Etkin, A.; Wager, T.D. Functional neuroimaging of anxiety: A meta-analysis of emotional processing in PTSD, social anxiety disorder, and specific phobia. *Am. J. Psychiatry* **2007**, *164*, 1476–1488. [CrossRef]
141. Duncan, L.E.; Ratanatharathorn, A.; Aiello, A.E.; Almli, L.M.; Amstadter, A.B.; Ashley-Koch, A.E.; Baker, D.G.; Beckham, J.C.; Bierut, L.J.; Bisson, J.; et al. Largest GWAS of PTSD (n = 20,070) yields genetic overlap with schizophrenia and sex differences in heritability. *Mol. Psychiatry* **2018**, *23*, 666–673. [CrossRef]
142. Bachmann, A.W.; Sedgley, T.L.; Jackson, R.V.; Gibson, J.N.; Young, R.M.; Torpy, D.J. Glucocorticoid receptor polymorphisms and post-traumatic stress disorder. *Psychoneuroendocrinology* **2005**, *30*, 297–306. [CrossRef]
143. Hauer, D.; Weis, F.; Papassotiropoulos, A.; Schmoeckel, M.; Beiras-Fernandez, A.; Lieke, J.; Kaufmann, I.; Kirchhoff, F.; Vogeser, M.; Roozendaal, B.; et al. Relationship of a common polymorphism of the glucocorticoid receptor gene to traumatic memories and posttraumatic stress disorder in patients after intensive care therapy. *Crit. Care Med.* **2011**, *39*, 643–650. [CrossRef] [PubMed]
144. van Zuiden, M.; Geuze, E.; Willemen, H.L.; Vermetten, E.; Maas, M.; Heijnen, C.J.; Kavelaars, A. Pre-existing high glucocorticoid receptor number predicting development of posttraumatic stress symptoms after military deployment. *Am. J. Psychiatry* **2011**, *168*, 89–96. [CrossRef] [PubMed]
145. Xie, P.; Kranzler, H.R.; Poling, J.; Stein, M.B.; Anton, R.F.; Farrer, L.A.; Gelernter, J. Interaction of FKBP5 with childhood adversity on risk for post-traumatic stress disorder. *Neuropsychopharmacology* **2010**, *35*, 1684–1692. [CrossRef]
146. Yehuda, R.; Cai, G.; Golier, J.A.; Sarapas, C.; Galea, S.; Ising, M.; Rein, T.; Schmeidler, J.; Muller-Myhsok, B.; Holsboer, F.; et al. Gene expression patterns associated with posttraumatic stress disorder following exposure to the World Trade Center attacks. *Biol. Psychiatry* **2009**, *66*, 708–711. [CrossRef] [PubMed]
147. Sarapas, C.; Cai, G.; Bierer, L.M.; Golier, J.A.; Galea, S.; Ising, M.; Rein, T.; Schmeidler, J.; Muller-Myhsok, B.; Uhr, M.; et al. Genetic markers for PTSD risk and resilience among survivors of the World Trade Center attacks. *Dis. Markers* **2011**, *30*, 101–110. [CrossRef] [PubMed]
148. van Zuiden, M.; Heijnen, C.J.; Maas, M.; Amarouchi, K.; Vermetten, E.; Geuze, E.; Kavelaars, A. Glucocorticoid sensitivity of leukocytes predicts PTSD, depressive and fatigue symptoms after military deployment: A prospective study. *Psychoneuroendocrinology* **2012**, *37*, 1822–1836. [CrossRef]
149. Boscarino, J.A.; Erlich, P.M.; Hoffman, S.N.; Zhang, X. Higher FKBP5, COMT, CHRNA5, and CRHR1 allele burdens are associated with PTSD and interact with trauma exposure: Implications for neuropsychiatric research and treatment. *Neuropsychiatr. Dis. Treat.* **2012**, *8*, 131–139. [CrossRef]
150. Mehta, D.; Gonik, M.; Klengel, T.; Rex-Haffner, M.; Menke, A.; Rubel, J.; Mercer, K.B.; Putz, B.; Bradley, B.; Holsboer, F.; et al. Using polymorphisms in FKBP5 to define biologically distinct subtypes of posttraumatic stress disorder: Evidence from endocrine and gene expression studies. *Arch. Gen. Psychiatry* **2011**, *68*, 901–910. [CrossRef]
151. Zhang, L.; Hu, X.Z.; Yu, T.; Chen, Z.; Dohl, J.; Li, X.; Benedek, D.M.; Fullerton, C.S.; Wynn, G.; Barrett, J.E.; et al. Genetic association of FKBP5 with PTSD in US service members deployed to Iraq and Afghanistan. *J. Psychiatr. Res.* **2020**, *122*, 48–53. [CrossRef]
152. Wang, Q.; Shelton, R.C.; Dwivedi, Y. Interaction between early-life stress and FKBP5 gene variants in major depressive disorder and post-traumatic stress disorder: A systematic review and meta-analysis. *J. Affect. Disord.* **2018**, *225*, 422–428. [CrossRef]
153. Wolf, E.J.; Mitchell, K.S.; Logue, M.W.; Baldwin, C.T.; Reardon, A.F.; Humphries, D.E.; Miller, M.W. Corticotropin releasing hormone receptor 2 (CRHR-2) gene is associated with decreased risk and severity of posttraumatic stress disorder in women. *Depress. Anxiety* **2013**, *30*, 1161–1169. [CrossRef] [PubMed]
154. Heim, C.; Newport, D.J.; Heit, S.; Graham, Y.P.; Wilcox, M.; Bonsall, R.; Miller, A.H.; Nemeroff, C.B. Pituitary-adrenal and autonomic responses to stress in women after sexual and physical abuse in childhood. *JAMA* **2000**, *284*, 592–597. [CrossRef] [PubMed]
155. Zannas, A.S.; Provencal, N.; Binder, E.B. Epigenetics of Posttraumatic Stress Disorder: Current Evidence, Challenges, and Future Directions. *Biol. Psychiatry* **2015**, *78*, 327–335. [CrossRef] [PubMed]

156. Watkeys, O.J.; Kremerskothen, K.; Quide, Y.; Fullerton, J.M.; Green, M.J. Glucocorticoid receptor gene (NR3C1) DNA methylation in association with trauma, psychopathology, transcript expression, or genotypic variation: A systematic review. *Neurosci. Biobehav. Rev.* **2018**, *95*, 85–122. [CrossRef]
157. Yehuda, R.; Flory, J.D.; Bierer, L.M.; Henn-Haase, C.; Lehrner, A.; Desarnaud, F.; Makotkine, I.; Daskalakis, N.P.; Marmar, C.R.; Meaney, M.J. Lower methylation of glucocorticoid receptor gene promoter 1F in peripheral blood of veterans with posttraumatic stress disorder. *Biol. Psychiatry* **2015**, *77*, 356–364. [CrossRef]
158. Vukojevic, V.; Kolassa, I.T.; Fastenrath, M.; Gschwind, L.; Spalek, K.; Milnik, A.; Heck, A.; Vogler, C.; Wilker, S.; Demougin, P.; et al. Epigenetic modification of the glucocorticoid receptor gene is linked to traumatic memory and post-traumatic stress disorder risk in genocide survivors. *J. Neurosci. Off. J. Soc. Neurosci.* **2014**, *34*, 10274–10284. [CrossRef]
159. Perroud, N.; Rutembesa, E.; Paoloni-Giacobino, A.; Mutabaruka, J.; Mutesa, L.; Stenz, L.; Malafosse, A.; Karege, F. The Tutsi genocide and transgenerational transmission of maternal stress: Epigenetics and biology of the HPA axis. *World J. Biol. Psychiatry* **2014**, *15*, 334–345. [CrossRef]
160. Labonte, B.; Azoulay, N.; Yerko, V.; Turecki, G.; Brunet, A. Epigenetic modulation of glucocorticoid receptors in posttraumatic stress disorder. *Transl. Psychiatry* **2014**, *4*, e368. [CrossRef]
161. Schechter, D.S.; Moser, D.A.; Paoloni-Giacobino, A.; Stenz, L.; Gex-Fabry, M.; Aue, T.; Adouan, W.; Cordero, M.I.; Suardi, F.; Manini, A.; et al. Methylation of NR3C1 is related to maternal PTSD, parenting stress and maternal medial prefrontal cortical activity in response to child separation among mothers with histories of violence exposure. *Front. Psychol.* **2015**, *6*, 690. [CrossRef]
162. Yehuda, R.; Daskalakis, N.P.; Bierer, L.M.; Bader, H.N.; Klengel, T.; Holsboer, F.; Binder, E.B. Holocaust Exposure Induced Intergenerational Effects on FKBP5 Methylation. *Biol. Psychiatry* **2016**, *80*, 372–380. [CrossRef]
163. Kang, J.I.; Kim, T.Y.; Choi, J.H.; So, H.S.; Kim, S.J. Allele-specific DNA methylation level of FKBP5 is associated with post-traumatic stress disorder. *Psychoneuroendocrinology* **2019**, *103*, 1–7. [CrossRef] [PubMed]
164. Lebow, M.A.; Schroeder, M.; Tsoory, M.; Holzman-Karniel, D.; Mehta, D.; Ben-Dor, S.; Gil, S.; Bradley, B.; Smith, A.K.; Jovanovic, T.; et al. Glucocorticoid-induced leucine zipper "quantifies" stressors and increases male susceptibility to PTSD. *Transl. Psychiatry* **2019**, *9*, 178. [CrossRef] [PubMed]
165. Rutten, B.P.F.; Vermetten, E.; Vinkers, C.H.; Ursini, G.; Daskalakis, N.P.; Pishva, E.; de Nijs, L.; Houtepen, L.C.; Eijssen, L.; Jaffe, A.E.; et al. Longitudinal analyses of the DNA methylome in deployed military servicemen identify susceptibility loci for post-traumatic stress disorder. *Mol. Psychiatry* **2018**, *23*, 1145–1156. [CrossRef] [PubMed]
166. Mehta, D.; Voisey, J.; Bruenig, D.; Harvey, W.; Morris, C.P.; Lawford, B.; Young, R.M. Transcriptome analysis reveals novel genes and immune networks dysregulated in veterans with PTSD. *Brainbehav. Immun.* **2018**, *74*, 133–142. [CrossRef] [PubMed]
167. Kumsta, R.; Marzi, S.J.; Viana, J.; Dempster, E.L.; Crawford, B.; Rutter, M.; Mill, J.; Sonuga-Barke, E.J. Severe psychosocial deprivation in early childhood is associated with increased DNA methylation across a region spanning the transcription start site of CYP2E1. *Transl. Psychiatry* **2016**, *6*, e830. [CrossRef] [PubMed]
168. Tylee, D.S.; Kawaguchi, D.M.; Glatt, S.J. On the outside, looking in: A review and evaluation of the comparability of blood and brain "-omes". *Am. J. Med. Genet. B Neuropsychiatr. Genet.* **2013**, *162B*, 595–603. [CrossRef]
169. Szyf, M.; Bick, J. DNA methylation: A mechanism for embedding early life experiences in the genome. *Child. Dev.* **2013**, *84*, 49–57. [CrossRef]
170. Schelling, G.; Briegel, J.; Roozendaal, B.; Stoll, C.; Rothenhausler, H.B.; Kapfhammer, H.P. The effect of stress doses of hydrocortisone during septic shock on posttraumatic stress disorder in survivors. *Biol. Psychiatry* **2001**, *50*, 978–985. [CrossRef]
171. Schelling, G.; Kilger, E.; Roozendaal, B.; de Quervain, D.J.; Briegel, J.; Dagge, A.; Rothenhausler, H.B.; Krauseneck, T.; Nollert, G.; Kapfhammer, H.P. Stress doses of hydrocortisone, traumatic memories, and symptoms of posttraumatic stress disorder in patients after cardiac surgery: A randomized study. *Biol. Psychiatry* **2004**, *55*, 627–633. [CrossRef]
172. Schelling, G.; Roozendaal, B.; Krauseneck, T.; Schmoelz, M.; De Quervain, D.; Briegel, J. Efficacy of hydrocortisone in preventing posttraumatic stress disorder following critical illness and major surgery. *Ann. NY Acad. Sci.* **2006**, *1071*, 46–53. [CrossRef]

173. Zohar, J.; Yahalom, H.; Kozlovsky, N.; Cwikel-Hamzany, S.; Matar, M.A.; Kaplan, Z.; Yehuda, R.; Cohen, H. High dose hydrocortisone immediately after trauma may alter the trajectory of PTSD: Interplay between clinical and animal studies. *Eur. Neuropsychopharmacol.* **2011**, *21*, 796–809. [CrossRef] [PubMed]
174. Delahanty, D.L.; Gabert-Quillen, C.; Ostrowski, S.A.; Nugent, N.R.; Fischer, B.; Morris, A.; Pitman, R.K.; Bon, J.; Fallon, W. The efficacy of initial hydrocortisone administration at preventing posttraumatic distress in adult trauma patients: A randomized trial. *CNS Spectr.* **2013**, *18*, 103–111. [CrossRef] [PubMed]
175. Aerni, A.; Traber, R.; Hock, C.; Roozendaal, B.; Schelling, G.; Papassotiropoulos, A.; Nitsch, R.M.; Schnyder, U.; de Quervain, D.J. Low-dose cortisol for symptoms of posttraumatic stress disorder. *Am. J. Psychiatry* **2004**, *161*, 1488–1490. [CrossRef] [PubMed]
176. Dunlop, B.W.; Binder, E.B.; Iosifescu, D.; Mathew, S.J.; Neylan, T.C.; Pape, J.C.; Carrillo-Roa, T.; Green, C.; Kinkead, B.; Grigoriadis, D.; et al. Corticotropin-Releasing Factor Receptor 1 Antagonism Is Ineffective for Women With Posttraumatic Stress Disorder. *Biol. Psychiatry* **2017**, *82*, 866–874. [CrossRef] [PubMed]
177. Ludascher, P.; Schmahl, C.; Feldmann, R.E., Jr.; Kleindienst, N.; Schneider, M.; Bohus, M. No evidence for differential dose effects of hydrocortisone on intrusive memories in female patients with complex post-traumatic stress disorder—A randomized, double-blind, placebo-controlled, crossover study. *J. Psychopharmacol.* **2015**, *29*, 1077–1084. [CrossRef] [PubMed]
178. Golier, J.A.; Yehuda, R.; Baker, D. A randomized clinical trial of a glucocorticoid receptor antagonist in PTSD. *Psychoneuroendocrinology* **2017**, *83*, 87. [CrossRef]
179. Yehuda, R.; Bierer, L.M.; Pratchett, L.C.; Lehrner, A.; Koch, E.C.; Van Manen, J.A.; Flory, J.D.; Makotkine, I.; Hildebrandt, T. Cortisol augmentation of a psychological treatment for warfighters with posttraumatic stress disorder: Randomized trial showing improved treatment retention and outcome. *Psychoneuroendocrinology* **2015**, *51*, 589–597. [CrossRef]
180. Galatzer-Levy, I.R.; Andero, R.; Sawamura, T.; Jovanovic, T.; Papini, S.; Ressler, K.J.; Norrholm, S.D. A cross species study of heterogeneity in fear extinction learning in relation to FKBP5 variation and expression: Implications for the acute treatment of posttraumatic stress disorder. *Neuropharmacology* **2017**, *116*, 188–195. [CrossRef]
181. Pape, J.C.; Carrillo-Roa, T.; Rothbaum, B.O.; Nemeroff, C.B.; Czamara, D.; Zannas, A.S.; Iosifescu, D.; Mathew, S.J.; Neylan, T.C.; Mayberg, H.S.; et al. DNA methylation levels are associated with CRF1 receptor antagonist treatment outcome in women with post-traumatic stress disorder. *Clin. Epigenet.* **2018**, *10*, 136. [CrossRef]
182. Ostacher, M.J.; Cifu, A.S. Management of Posttraumatic Stress Disorder. *JAMA* **2019**, *321*, 200–201. [CrossRef]
183. Watkins, L.E.; Sprang, K.R.; Rothbaum, B.O. Treating PTSD: A Review of Evidence-Based Psychotherapy Interventions. *Front. Behav. Neurosci.* **2018**, *12*, 258. [CrossRef] [PubMed]
184. Brom, D.; Kleber, R.J.; Defares, P.B. Brief psychotherapy for posttraumatic stress disorders. *J. Consult. Clin. Psychol.* **1989**, *57*, 607–612. [CrossRef] [PubMed]
185. Gerber, A.J.; Kocsis, J.H.; Milrod, B.L.; Roose, S.P.; Barber, J.P.; Thase, M.E.; Perkins, P.; Leon, A.C. A quality-based review of randomized controlled trials of psychodynamic psychotherapy. *Am. J. Psychiatry* **2011**, *168*, 19–28. [CrossRef] [PubMed]
186. Thoma, N.C.; McKay, D.; Gerber, A.J.; Milrod, B.L.; Edwards, A.R.; Kocsis, J.H. A quality-based review of randomized controlled trials of cognitive-behavioral therapy for depression: An assessment and metaregression. *Am. J. Psychiatry* **2012**, *169*, 22–30. [CrossRef] [PubMed]
187. Cordioli, A.V. As principais psicoterapias: Fundamentos teóricos, técnicas, indicações e contra-indicações. In *Psicoterapias: Abordagens Atuais*, 3rd ed.; Cordioli, A.V., Ed.; Artmed Editora S.A.: Porto Alegre, Brazil, 2008; pp. 19–41.
188. Lambert, M.J. Outcome in psychotherapy: The past and important advances. *Psychotherapy* **2013**, *50*, 42–51. [CrossRef] [PubMed]
189. Roth, A.; Fonagy, P. *What Works for Whom? A Critical Review of Psychotherapy Research*, 2nd ed.; Guilford Press: New York, NY, USA, 2005.
190. Daskalakis, N.P.; Bagot, R.C.; Parker, K.J.; Vinkers, C.H.; de Kloet, E.R. The three-hit concept of vulnerability and resilience: Toward understanding adaptation to early-life adversity outcome. *Psychoneuroendocrinology* **2013**, *38*, 1858–1873. [CrossRef] [PubMed]
191. Nederhof, E.; Schmidt, M.V. Mismatch or cumulative stress: Toward an integrated hypothesis of programming effects. *Physiol. Behav.* **2012**, *106*, 691–700. [CrossRef] [PubMed]

192. Yehuda, R.; LeDoux, J. Response variation following trauma: A translational neuroscience approach to understanding PTSD. *Neuron* **2007**, *56*, 19–32. [CrossRef]
193. Meir Drexler, S.; Wolf, O.T. The role of glucocorticoids in emotional memory reconsolidation. *Neurobiol. Learn. Mem.* **2017**, *142*, 126–134. [CrossRef]
194. Rapcencu, A.E.; Gorter, R.; Kennis, M.; van Rooij, S.J.H.; Geuze, E. Pre-treatment cortisol awakening response predicts symptom reduction in posttraumatic stress disorder after treatment. *Psychoneuroendocrinology* **2017**, *82*, 1–8. [CrossRef]
195. Rauch, S.A.; King, A.P.; Abelson, J.; Tuerk, P.W.; Smith, E.; Rothbaum, B.O.; Clifton, E.; Defever, A.; Liberzon, I. Biological and symptom changes in posttraumatic stress disorder treatment: A randomized clinical trial. *Depress. Anxiety* **2015**, *32*, 204–212. [CrossRef] [PubMed]
196. Dajani, R.; Hadfield, K.; van Uum, S.; Greff, M.; Panter-Brick, C. Hair cortisol concentrations in war-affected adolescents: A prospective intervention trial. *Psychoneuroendocrinology* **2018**, *89*, 138–146. [CrossRef] [PubMed]
197. Steudte-Schmiedgen, S.; Kirschbaum, C.; Alexander, N.; Stalder, T. An integrative model linking traumatization, cortisol dysregulation and posttraumatic stress disorder: Insight from recent hair cortisol findings. *Neurosci. Biobehav. Rev.* **2016**, *69*, 124–135. [CrossRef] [PubMed]
198. Roozendaal, B.; Hahn, E.L.; Nathan, S.V.; de Quervain, D.J.; McGaugh, J.L. Glucocorticoid effects on memory retrieval require concurrent noradrenergic activity in the hippocampus and basolateral amygdala. *J. Neurosci. Off. J. Soc. Neurosci.* **2004**, *24*, 8161–8169. [CrossRef] [PubMed]
199. de Quervain, D.J.; Aerni, A.; Schelling, G.; Roozendaal, B. Glucocorticoids and the regulation of memory in health and disease. *Front. Neuroendocr.* **2009**, *30*, 358–370. [CrossRef]
200. Quide, Y.; Witteveen, A.B.; El-Hage, W.; Veltman, D.J.; Olff, M. Differences between effects of psychological versus pharmacological treatments on functional and morphological brain alterations in anxiety disorders and major depressive disorder: A systematic review. *Neurosci. Biobehav. Rev.* **2012**, *36*, 626–644. [CrossRef]
201. Butler, O.; Willmund, G.; Gleich, T.; Gallinat, J.; Kuhn, S.; Zimmermann, P. Hippocampal gray matter increases following multimodal psychological treatment for combat-related post-traumatic stress disorder. *Brain Behav.* **2018**, *8*, e00956. [CrossRef]
202. Sapolsky, R.M.; Romero, L.M.; Munck, A.U. How do glucocorticoids influence stress responses? Integrating permissive, suppressive, stimulatory, and preparative actions. *Endocr. Rev.* **2000**, *21*, 55–89. [CrossRef]
203. Eriksson, P.S.; Perfilieva, E.; Bjork-Eriksson, T.; Alborn, A.M.; Nordborg, C.; Peterson, D.A.; Gage, F.H. Neurogenesis in the adult human hippocampus. *Nat. Med.* **1998**, *4*, 1313–1317. [CrossRef]
204. Margraf, J.; Zlomuzica, A. Changing the future, not the past: A translational paradigm shift in treating anxiety. *EMBO Rep.* **2015**, *16*, 259–260. [CrossRef]
205. Kandel, E.R. A new intellectual framework for psychiatry. *Am. J. Psychiatry* **1998**, *155*, 457–469. [CrossRef] [PubMed]
206. Hauer, D.; Kolassa, I.T.; Laubender, R.P.; Mansmann, U.; Hagl, C.; Roozendaal, B.; de Quervain, D.J.; Schelling, G. A genotype-specific, randomized controlled behavioral intervention to improve the neuroemotional outcome of cardiac surgery: Study protocol for a randomized controlled trial. *Trials* **2013**, *14*, 89. [CrossRef] [PubMed]
207. Vinkers, C.; Geuze, E.; van Rooij, S.; Kennis, M.; Schur, R.; Nispeling, D.; Smith, A.; Nievergelt, C.; Uddin, M.; Rutten, B.; et al. O41. Longitudinal Changes in Genome-Wide DNA Methylation Levels Related to Treatment Outcomes and Recovery From Post-Traumatic Stress Disorder. *Biol. Psychiatry* **2019**, *85*, S122–S123. [CrossRef]
208. Jakobsson, J.; Cordero, M.I.; Bisaz, R.; Groner, A.C.; Busskamp, V.; Bensadoun, J.C.; Cammas, F.; Losson, R.; Mansuy, I.M.; Sandi, C.; et al. KAP1-mediated epigenetic repression in the forebrain modulates behavioral vulnerability to stress. *Neuron* **2008**, *60*, 818–831. [CrossRef]
209. Feodorova, Y.N.; Sarafian, V.S. Psychological stress—cellular and molecular mechanisms. *Folia Med. (Plovdiv)* **2012**, *54*, 5–13. [CrossRef] [PubMed]
210. Zerach, G.; Kanat-Maymon, Y.; Aloni, R.; Solomon, Z. The role of fathers' psychopathology in the intergenerational transmission of captivity trauma: A twenty three-year longitudinal study. *J. Affect. Disord.* **2016**, *190*, 84–92. [CrossRef] [PubMed]
211. Lang, A.J.; Gartstein, M.A. Intergenerational transmission of traumatization: Theoretical framework and implications for prevention. *J. Trauma Dissociation Off. J. Int. Soc. Study Dissociation* **2018**, *19*, 162–175. [CrossRef] [PubMed]

212. Gentile, S. Early pregnancy exposure to selective serotonin reuptake inhibitors, risks of major structural malformations, and hypothesized teratogenic mechanisms. *Exp. Opin. Drug Metab. Toxicol.* **2015**, *11*, 1585–1597. [CrossRef]
213. Tomaz, T.; Castro-Vale, I. Trauma-Informed Care in Primary Health Settings-Which Is Even More Needed in Times of COVID-19. *Healthcare (Basel)* **2020**, *8*, 340. [CrossRef]

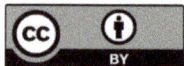

© 2020 by the authors. Licensee MDPI, Basel, Switzerland. This article is an open access article distributed under the terms and conditions of the Creative Commons Attribution (CC BY) license (http://creativecommons.org/licenses/by/4.0/).

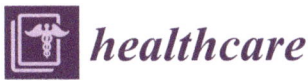

Article

Vulnerability Factors Associated with Lifetime Posttraumatic Stress Disorder among Veterans 40 Years after War

Ivone Castro-Vale [1],*, Milton Severo [2], Davide Carvalho [3] and Rui Mota-Cardoso [4]

1. Medical Psychology Unit, Department of Clinical Neurosciences and Mental Health, Faculty of Medicine, University of Porto, 4200-319 Porto, Portugal
2. Department of Clinical Epidemiology, Predictive Medicine and Public Health, and Department of Medical Education and Simulation, Faculty of Medicine, University of Porto, 4200-319 Porto, Portugal; milton@med.up.pt
3. Department of Endocrinology, Diabetes and Metabolism, São João Hospital University Centre, Faculty of Medicine, University of Porto, 4200-319 Porto, Portugal; davideccarvalho@gmail.com
4. i3S-Institute for Research and Innovation in Health, University of Porto, 4200-135 Porto, Portugal; rmc@med.up.pt

* Correspondence: ivonecastrovale@med.up.pt; Tel.: +351-22-0426920

Received: 14 August 2020; Accepted: 22 September 2020; Published: 24 September 2020

Abstract: Vulnerability factors for posttraumatic stress disorder (PTSD) development are still controversial. Our aim was to study the vulnerability factors for the development of war-related PTSD over a period of 40 years after exposure. A cross-sectional, observational study was carried out on 61 male traumatized war veterans, taking into consideration adverse childhood experiences (ACE), attachment orientations, number of non-war-related traumatic events, and war experiences. Lifetime PTSD was assessed by using the Clinician-Administered PTSD Scale. Insecure attachment styles were significantly associated with lifetime PTSD and even after adjustment for war exposure this was still significant. Non-war-related traumatic events were not associated with lifetime PTSD, whereas ACE were associated with lifetime PTSD. War-related experiences were also associated with lifetime PTSD, except for injury or disease. The results for our sample show that, 40 years after war, the intensity of war-related experiences and ACE were significantly and independently associated with the development of lifetime PTSD. Insecure attachment was significantly associated with lifetime PTSD, which, in turn, are both positively associated with war exposure. These findings may have implications for patient care, as they constitute a strong argument that attachment-focused therapies could well be necessary 40 years after trauma.

Keywords: posttraumatic stress disorder; war veterans; trauma and stressor related disorders; adverse childhood experiences; attachment

1. Introduction

Posttraumatic stress disorder (PTSD) diagnostic criteria have recently been reviewed in the fifth edition of the Diagnostic and Statistical Manual of Mental Disorders (DSM-5) [1]. PTSD diagnosis requires the experience of a traumatic event (TE) to bring on its development. The TE definition has also changed from DSM-IV to DSM-5 criteria, with the latter not requiring the person to feel intense fear, helplessness, or horror—as DSM-IV does. It has been estimated that 9.2% of those exposed to a TE will have PTSD [2]. The reason why only a minority of exposed people come to develop PTSD is the focus of much research. Vulnerability factors have been described and can be grouped into three clusters. Pre-traumatic vulnerability factors have been found, such as: arousal, negative affect, hostility, anger, lower cognitive abilities, psychopathology, prior trauma, poor family functioning, poverty, and a family history of psychopathology. Among perceived peritraumatic vulnerability factors, life stress, emotional responses, and dissociation have all been found to predict PTSD development. Finally, it was found that lack of social support was the main posttrauma vulnerability factor for predicting PTSD development [3,4]. It has been found that peritraumatic factors are more predictive of posttraumatic growth, whilst pretrauma and personality-related variables are only predictive of PTSD [5]. Out of the personality variables, avoidant attachment significantly contributed to variance in PTSD risk.

Attachment is a construct which is related to the pattern of relationships established by a person with significant others. Attachment starts with the first relationships established between children and their caretakers, and is shaped by other relationships and events throughout the life cycle [6]. Attachment security influences the way a person copes with adversities and stress through positive mental representations of self and others [7]. On the other hand, insecure attachment orientations (anxiety and/or avoidance) predispose a person to mental disorders, due to the absence of a stable mental organization [7,8]. Attachment orientation predicts how adults react to stress and TEs [9,10]. Some studies suggest that attachment patterns moderate the association between TEs and PTSD [11,12]. Several attachment-related TEs are characterized by high conditional risk for PTSD development, or cause high PTSD burden to society, such as the sudden unexpected death of a loved one, war, sexual violence, and witnessing atrocities [2,13–15]. Furthermore, trauma severity has also been found to moderate the association between attachment and PTSD [16]. O'Connor and Elklit [17] found a negative correlation between secure attachment and PTSD symptoms when studying a non-clinical population, which suggested that secure attachment protects against the development of PTSD. This was also found in the case of combat-related PTSD [18,19]. On the other hand, PTSD was shown to influence attachment insecurity [20,21]. Furthermore, attachment has been shown to be negatively influenced by maltreatment as a child [22]. Attachment orientations can be studied as pretraumatic vulnerability factors for PTSD development, but also as peritraumatic, and even as a consequence of the disorder itself.

Among the pretraumatic vulnerability factors, adverse childhood experiences (ACE) have been related to the development of PTSD, with an increase of risk after exposure to the index TE [23]. Childhood adversities can challenge secure attachment organizations and have enduring consequences on attachment orientations and psychopathology [24,25]. ACE have also been associated with combat-related PTSD, particularly in the case of physical neglect and multiple types of adversities [26].

Different TEs are related to different incidence rates of PTSD, the highest rates being related to interpersonal violence [2]. War-related TEs are well-known risk factors for the development of PTSD, as well as traumatic load [27,28]. Specific combat experiences are associated with different risks to develop PTSD [29,30]. Some of these war experiences, such as atrocities and killing, may constitute severe transgressions of combatants' deepest moral standards, and cause what Litz et al. [31] defined as 'moral injury'—the long-term negative consequences at psychological, behavioral, religious, emotional, biological, and social levels. The study of war-related PTSD demands that war experiences are well characterized. However, the results regarding the influence of attachment orientations in the relationship between TEs and PTSD development are conflicting [9,11].

Portugal was involved in a war conflict from 1961 to 1974 with Angola, Mozambique, and Portuguese Guinea (currently Guinea-Bissau), which were former colonies fighting for their independence. Most of the soldiers were deployed non-voluntarily for a period of 24 months of guerrilla war.

Portuguese veterans of the colonial wars have a high prevalence (39%) of probable PTSD [32]. In addition, the time lapse of 40 years after the end of these wars provides a long after-trauma period for PTSD to develop, including delayed onset—a subtype of PTSD which applies to those cases when symptoms only begin six months or more after exposure to the TE [33]. Nevertheless, only a few studies have researched this population. Furthermore, the number of older war veterans is rising and, as the majority retain their diagnosis of PTSD following evidence-based interventions, and one third drop out of treatment, it is therefore important to characterize this population further [34]. The aim of this study was to investigate some of the vulnerability factors for lifetime PTSD development, over a period of 40 years after war-related TE, in a sample of Portuguese war veterans, especially focusing on ACE, attachment orientations, war experiences, and the experience of non-war-related TEs. In addition, we studied whether the association between war exposure and lifetime PTSD was confounded by or interacted with attachment orientations.

2. Materials and Methods

2.1. General Procedure

This cross-sectional, observational research is part of a larger study on the neurobiological inheritance of PTSD, which was approved by the Ethics Committee of our University (Comissão de Ética para a Saúde do Centro Hospitalar de São João/Faculdade de Medicina da Universidade do Porto, approval number: CES-138/08). Having received a complete written and verbal description of the study, all the participants gave their written informed consent. Interaction with the participants was carried out in a university setting and was solely performed by the same researcher and was carried out individually during one appointment. No financial compensation was paid for participating in this study, although payment for transport to the university was provided.

2.2. Participants

We used two ways of selecting participants (for a detailed description see Castro-Vale et al. [35]): 75.4% were from an outpatient clinic of the Portuguese Disabled Veterans Association (ADFA), and 24.6% were from three lists of war veterans' companies from war time. Sixty-one male, Caucasian veterans (mean age of 65.25 (range = 60–74, SD = 3.37 years)) from the Portuguese colonial wars agreed to participate.

Participants with and without lifetime PTSD were included if they fulfilled the war-related DSM-IV [36] criterion A for PTSD, and also if they had children (as this is part of a larger study on the neurobiological intergenerational transmission of PTSD). The general exclusion criteria for participants were the following: the presence of neurologic, infectious, or any active medical illness, and any DSM-IV psychotic, bipolar, or neurocognitive disorders. Participants with lifetime PTSD were also excluded if they had current substance-related disorders. The specific exclusion criteria for the war veterans' group without PTSD were the following: if they had ever had PTSD and if they also had any current psychiatric disorder.

2.3. Measures

The Graffar Index was used to measure the socioeconomic status (SES) [37,38]. This Index classifies subjects into five classes, with 1 being the highest, and 5 the lowest SES class. The clinical history and other sociodemographic data were also collected.

The Clinician-Administered PTSD Scale (CAPS) [39] was used to characterize the participants in relation to PTSD diagnosis, and also to research the lifetime number and the type of TEs experienced. Lifetime PTSD was considered if participants had DSM-IV criteria, in accordance with Blake et al.'s [40] rule (frequency ≥ 1 and intensity ≥ 2) and a total CAPS score of 50 or more. TEs were assessed with the CAPS Life Events Checklist and were subsequently checked for DSM-IV A2 criterion, following the CAPS procedure. TEs occurring before and after the war were counted separately from each other, and also from war-related TEs. In our sample, the Cronbach's alpha (reliability) of the CAPS was superior to 0.90.

To determine participants' eligibility requirements for the study, current and past psychiatric disorders where investigated, using the Structured Clinical Interview for DSM-IV axis I (SCID-I) [41] except for the PTSD module.

The Childhood Trauma Questionnaire-Short Form (CTQ-SF) [42,43] is a retrospective, self-reported questionnaire which contains 28 questions about specific maltreatment experiences during childhood and adolescence. The items are classified into a 5-point ordinal scale, according to the frequency of exposure to that specific experience. The Total CTQ-SF score provides a general ACE score, and not just TEs. It also provides scores for five different types of maltreatment, namely: emotional abuse; physical abuse; sexual abuse; emotional neglect, and; physical neglect.

Attachment style was studied with the Revised Adult Attachment Scale (RAAS) [44,45]. This scale consists of 18 items, which were scored on a 5-point Likert scale. The scale contains three dimensions: anxiety, close, and depend. The close and depend dimensions are positively correlated and can be gathered as close–depend. Close and depend dimensions were averaged and were then reverse scored to yield the attachment-related avoidance dimension. According to the scores obtained for each dimension, Bartholomew's [46] attachment styles classification was adopted, namely: secure, dismissing, preoccupied, and fearful. These attachment styles are described as follows (adapted from [44]): secure—those participants who scored an average score below the midpoint (3.0) on avoidance, and below or equal to the midpoint on anxiety; dismissing—those whose scoring was above or equal to the midpoint on avoidance, and below or equal to the midpoint on anxiety; preoccupied—those scoring below the midpoint on avoidance, and above the midpoint on anxiety; fearful—those scoring above or equal to the midpoint on avoidance, and above the midpoint on anxiety. Those participants with dismissing, preoccupied, and fearful styles were also grouped in the insecure style [47].

In order to characterize and quantify the different war-related experiences of the veterans, we constructed the War Exposure Questionnaire (WEQ; see Supplementary Materials)—which was adapted to the specificities of the guerrilla war where each veteran fought. This questionnaire was adapted from the "Severity of Exposure Index", which was used for the same purpose [32]. The WEQ has 38 items, which inquire about eight different subdomains of war-related experiences (war-related experiences, physical conditions, injury or disease, witnessing casualties amongst comrades, witnessing casualties amongst the enemy, witnessing casualties amongst civilians, actions on the enemy, and action against civilians). Each sub-domain is the result of the sum of positively-answered questions (e.g., have you been tortured?) which are related to that subject. The total sum provides a total WEQ score (ranging from 0 to 38), which represents war exposure, and which was used as a surrogate for war severity. In our sample, the Cronbach's alpha (reliability) of the total WEQ score was 0.81.

2.4. Statistical Methods

The chi-square test, or the Fisher exact test was used to test the association between qualitative variables. The two independent sample *t*-test was used to compare the quantitative variables.

Odds ratio and the respective 95% CI was used to estimate the magnitude of the association between lifetime PTSD and several vulnerability factors. Simple and multinomial unconditional logistic regression was used to estimate the crude and adjusted odds ratio. The interaction between independent variables with lifetime PTSD was studied using logistic regression models.

3. Results

Participant's characteristics are depicted in Table 1. Groups with, and without lifetime PTSD are identical with regards the subjects' age, marital status, prevalence of disability, Graffar classification, and the deployment site where they were at war. All the veterans self-reported good physical and mental health before going to war.

Table 1. Sociodemographic characteristics of the total sample and according to having or not having lifetime PTSD.

Sociodemographic Characteristic	Total (n = 61)	PTSD (n = 33)	Non-PTSD (n = 28)	p
Age, Years (Mean, SD)	65.25, 3.37	64.82, 3.41	65.75, 3.30	0.285
Marital Status	N (%)	N (%)	N (%)	
Married	57 (93.4)	32 (97.0)	25 (89.3)	0.325
Divorced or Widow	4 (6.6)	1 (3.0)	3 (10.7)	
Graffar Index				
2	8 (13.1)	2 (6.1)	6 (21.4)	0.082
3	38 (62.3)	20 (60.6)	18 (64.3)	
4	15 (24.6)	11 (33.3)	4 (14.3)	
Disability				
No	38 (62.3)	23 (69.6)	15 (53.6)	0.195
Yes	23 (37.7)	10 (30.3)	13 (46.4)	
Territory (Deployment Site)				
Angola	22 (36.1)	11 (33.3)	11 (39.3)	0.484
Mozambique	19 (31.1)	9 (27.3)	10 (35.7)	
Guinea	20 (32.8)	13 (39.4)	7 (25.0)	

Note: PTSD, posttraumatic stress disorder.

Attachment was significantly associated with lifetime PTSD (Table 2). High scores in anxiety and avoidance attachment were significantly associated with lifetime PTSD ($p = 0.002$ and 0.001, respectively). The association between anxiety and lifetime PTSD ceased to exist when adjusting for avoidance and total war exposure (total WEQ score). On the other hand, the association between avoidance and lifetime PTSD was attenuated, but still significant when adjusting for anxiety and total war exposure ($OR = 7.21$; 95% CI 1.02, 50.94; Table 2). When dimensions were converted to attachment styles, the prevalence of lifetime PTSD was significantly different between groups ($p = 0.005$; Figure 1). The groups with the dismissing ($p = 0.040$) and fearful ($p = 0.004$) styles of attachment have a higher prevalence of lifetime PTSD than the secure style group. A significant association was found between insecure attachment styles and lifetime PTSD ($OR = 6.37$; 95% CI 1.81, 22.46; Table 2). When adjusting for total war exposure, the association between insecure attachment styles and lifetime PTSD was attenuated, but was still significant ($OR = 4.04$; 95% CI 1.00, 16.34).

Table 2. Association between attachment dimensions and non-war-related traumatic events and lifetime posttraumatic stress disorder—both crude and adjusted.

Attachment and TEs	Unadjusted OR (95% CI)	p	Adjusted OR (95% CI)	p
Attachment				
Anxiety	3.76 (1.66, 8.52)	0.002	2.34 (0.82, 6.65) [a]	0.111
Avoidance	18.46 (3.16, 107.72)	0.001	7.21 (1.02, 50.94) [a]	0.048
Total WEQ score	1.18 (1.07, 1.31)	<0.001	1.17 (1.04, 1.31) [a]	0.007
Insecure versus Secure	6.37 (1.81, 22.46)	0.002	4.04 (1.00, 16.34) [b]	0.043
TEs before War				
Yes versus no	0.52 (0.13, 2.09)	0.354	-	-
TEs after War				
Yes versus no	0.52 (0.19, 1.46)	0.211	-	-

Note: OR, odds ratio; CI, confidence interval; WEQ, War Exposure Questionnaire; TEs, traumatic events. [a] Model adjusted for attachment anxiety and avoidance and total WEQ score. [b] Adjusted for total war exposure.

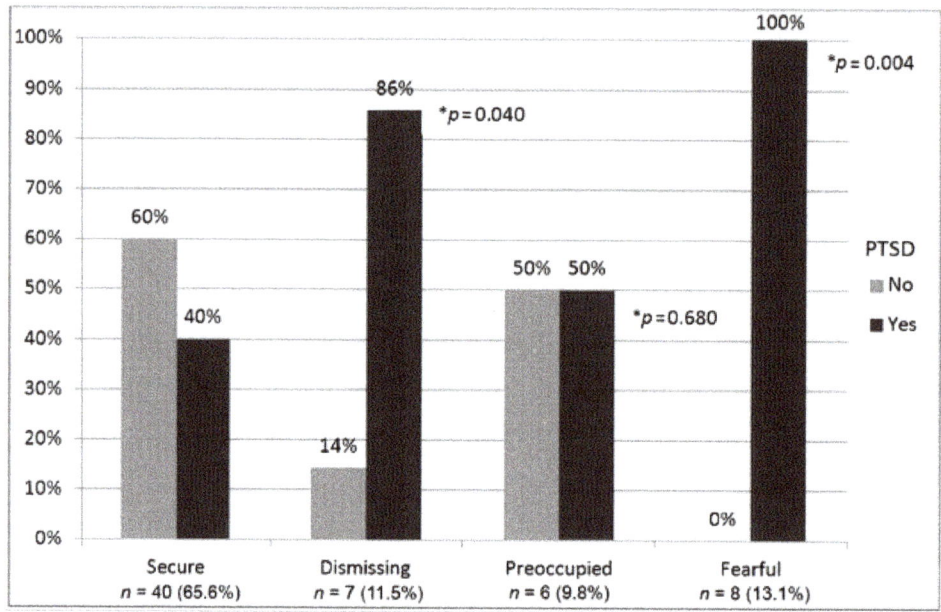

Figure 1. Prevalence of lifetime posttraumatic stress disorder (PTSD) by styles of attachment ($p = 0.005$).
* Considering as reference, the secure style.

Having experienced non-war-related TEs (either before or after the war) was not associated with lifetime PTSD (Table 2). ACE, as assessed by the CTQ-SF, showed that total CTQ-SF experiences ($p = 0.037$), and particularly, emotional abuse ($p = 0.024$) and physical neglect ($p = 0.004$) were significantly associated with lifetime PTSD development (Table 3). Total CTQ-SF experiences remained significantly associated with lifetime PTSD after adjustment for total war-related experiences ($p = 0.039$). Furthermore, total CTQ-SF experiences did not interact with total war experiences to predict lifetime PTSD (data not shown).

Table 3. Vulnerability factors for lifetime posttraumatic stress disorder development.

Vulnerability Factors	Crude OR (95% CI)	p	Adjusted OR (95% CI)	p
CTQ-SF				
Total CTQ-SF score	1.06 (1.00, 1.13)	0.037	1.07 (1.00, 1.15) [a]	0.039
Emotional abuse	1.27 (0.99, 1.63)	0.024	-	-
Emotional neglect	1.05 (0.93, 1.18)	0.454	-	-
Sexual abuse	0.72 (0.31, 1.69)	0.430	-	-
Physical abuse	1.1 (0.87, 1.39)	0.414	-	-
Physical neglect	1.23 (1.05, 1.44)	0.004	-	-
War-Related Experiences (WEQ)				
Total WEQ score	1.18 (1.07, 1.31)	<0.001	1.18 (1.07, 1.31) [b]	<0.001
War-related experiences	2.05 (1.18, 3.57)	0.004	-	-
Physical conditions	1.87 (1.15, 3.06)	0.005	-	-
Injury or disease	1.11 (0.80, 1.65)	0.462	-	-
Witnessing casualties amongst comrades	1.42 (0.99, 2.04)	0.045	-	-
Witnessing casualties amongst the enemy	1.59 (1.17, 2.16)	0.001	-	-
Witnessing casualties amongst civilians	1.74 (1.23, 2.47)	<0.001	-	-
Action against the enemy	2.03 (1.25, 3.28)	0.002	-	-

Note: OR, odds ratio; CI, confidence interval; CTQ-SF, Childhood Trauma Questionnaire-Short Form; WEQ, War Exposure Questionnaire. [a] Adjusted for total war-related experiences (total WEQ score). [b] Adjusted for total childhood adversities (total CTQ-SF score).

With regards to war-related experiences, these were all significantly associated with lifetime PTSD, except for the case of those related to injury or disease (Table 3). Adjusting total war-related experiences to childhood adversities did not change the OR (Table 3), nor did adjusting for attachment dimensions (Table 2). Furthermore, total war experiences did not interact with attachment dimensions to predict lifetime PTSD (data not shown). In relation to action against civilians, 25 (49%) of the subjects who did not report this experience developed lifetime PTSD, whilst the nine (100%) who did report this experience developed lifetime PTSD ($p = 0.013$).

4. Discussion

We found that attachment orientations were associated with lifetime PTSD, particularly the insecure attachment styles. When adjusted for war exposure, this association decreased, but was still present. This means that war exposure is a confounder of the association between attachment and PTSD, or in other words, war exposure is associated with attachment and also with lifetime PTSD.

According to the attachment theory, insecure attachment is a risk factor for the development and increase in PTSD symptoms. However, Solomon et al. [21] found that PTSD symptoms predict attachment patterns better than attachment predicts PTSD symptoms. On the other hand, a longitudinal study concluded that PTSD symptoms both influenced, and were influenced by, attachment patterns, and that attachment insecurity contributes to maintaining PTSD symptoms over time [20]. Recent cross-sectional studies have found associations between attachment styles and war-related PTSD, however the design of these studies does not permit one to draw conclusions on causality e.g., [18,19]. As our study does not also allow one to make conclusions about causality, longitudinal studies should be pursued in order to clarify these relationships further.

Considering Bartholomew's [46] styles, in our study, the group of participants with the secure attachment style had a lower prevalence of lifetime PTSD than those with dismissing and fearful styles. These findings are probably related with the high association that we found between the avoidance dimension and PTSD. Clark and Owens [18] also found that the highest association with PTSD symptom severity was for avoidance attachment. As they argue, attachment avoidance may have some overlap with the avoidant and numbing PTSD symptoms, and it has been suggested that these increase across time [48]. A recent meta-analysis of the relationship between adult attachment style and post-traumatic stress symptoms found a modest overall population effect size for avoidant attachment [49]. In our study, all participants with the fearful style had lifetime PTSD. Other studies have found fearful style to be associated with the highest scores for PTSD symptoms (e.g., [19,49]). Studies of non-clinical and non-war-related PTSD samples also found associations between attachment and PTSD symptoms [50]—particularly associations with the dismissing and fearful styles [17,51]. Furthermore, a recent meta-analysis found that the study design (cross-sectional, longitudinal, controlled comparison, or intervention) does not moderate the relationship between insecure attachment and overall PTSD symptoms [49].

Forty years after the war ended, veterans from the study sample with lifetime PTSD demonstrate insecure attachment patterns. This finding supports the argument that specific psychotherapeutic interventions focusing on attachment organization [52–54] should be pursued with these patients, as attachment orientation modification was evident in one PTSD sample after exposure psychotherapy [55]. Such interventions could have consequences both in modifying PTSD symptoms, and also for the formation of a therapeutic relationship, which is also important for recovery. Furthermore, the availability of improving psychotherapeutic interventions for PTSD patients of this age group, such as prolonged exposure therapy, is required—as treatment gains do not appear to be maintained at six-months follow-up [56,57]. Independently of the possible causal relationships between attachment and PTSD, existing studies show that attachment-focused therapeutic interventions can improve PTSD symptoms [58,59]. Additionally, an attachment-directed psychotherapy model has been proposed, which is supported by the relationship between war-related TEs and "moral injury" [53]. Furthermore, one study found that attachment style can predict treatment outcome, and thus improve our knowledge with regards to which psychotherapy works best for whom, and which can be more cost-effective [60]. However, more studies are needed to help us better understand how attachment-focused interventions can be used in clinical practice with PTSD patients.

In our research, we found that total childhood adversity, and particularly, emotional abuse and physical neglect were significantly associated with lifetime PTSD development assessed 40 years after war-related TEs. The association between total childhood adversities and PTSD development was independent of total war experiences.

Another recent cross-sectional study of veterans of the Portuguese colonial wars found that those with PTSD (recruited from the Psychiatry Department of one military hospital) reported significantly higher total ACE scores, and, specifically, a greater level of childhood emotional and physical abuse than those without PTSD (recruited from a snowball sample) [61]. A study of a representative sample of veterans of the same wars found low, but significant correlations between childhood abuse and neglect and PTSD symptoms [32].

Our findings are similar to those of a longitudinal study that assessed ACE before deployment to military conflicts, which found that those who reported ACE in more than one category were at an increased risk of developing post-deployment PTSD—with the strongest association being for physical neglect [26]. Other studies found that the number of childhood traumatic experiences was significantly higher in the group of participants who developed post-deployment PTSD symptoms [62] and that this significantly predicted a high level of PTSD symptoms [23]. ACE could be linked to the increased risk of PTSD development through negative influences on attachment orientations [22], among other causes.

We found that lifetime non-war-related TEs, either before or after war, were not associated with lifetime PTSD, which is contrary to the current belief that prior traumatization [4] and additional life stress [63] are risk factors for developing PTSD. Recent studies have found that prior experience of TEs in the absence of subsequent PTSD development is not a risk factor for PTSD development [64,65]. In our study, prior PTSD was not probable, as all the veterans self-reported good mental health before going to war.

In this study, we specifically assessed TEs as defined by criterion A of the DSM-IV PTSD diagnostic criteria. This criterion enables the evaluation of only those TEs that can cause PTSD, according to DSM-IV. Other studies use a much broader concept of traumatization [66]—or they simply do not define prior TE [67]. In addition, the meta-analysis of Ozer et al. [4] found that the relationship between prior trauma and PTSD was stronger if PTSD resulted from non-combat interpersonal violence, rather than if it resulted from combat exposure.

Combat-related trauma severity is a well-known risk factor for PTSD development [29,63]. We found that all types of war-related experiences were significantly positively associated with lifetime PTSD development, except for the case of war-related experiences of injury or disease. This finding is interesting, as this experience could represent a direct threat to life, although maybe this was experienced by the majority of war veterans, as it meant the end of the war for them. Different results were reported [28], which did not find that combat exposure increases the risk of developing PTSD symptoms, however certain specific war experiences did—such as being wounded or injured and killing an enemy. Further research of this subdomain is warranted, separating injury from disease.

Several recent longitudinal studies have shown similar results to our study. Carrying out a combat role during deployment was significantly associated with probable PTSD [68]. The frequency and intensity of combat were strong predictors of new-onset probable PTSD—specifically the experience of killing [29]. Rona et al. [30] found that combat exposure was a strong and specific predictor of PTSD—especially when involving close contact with the enemy.

In our study, action against civilians was significantly associated with lifetime PTSD development, which is a combat experience that has not been independently reported recently (e.g., [29,30]). This is probably one of the war-related experiences which is most prone to cause moral injuries [31].

We found that attachment patterns did not confound or interact with the association between total war experiences and lifetime PTSD. Another study [9] did not find a moderation role for attachment in the association between intimate partner violence and PTSD, while another [11] did for the anxiety and depend dimensions, but not for the close dimension. These discrepancies could be due to the different methodologies and different TEs assessed. War experiences seem to be strong predictors for lifetime PTSD development in our sample, as they are neither influenced by attachment orientations, nor by childhood adversities.

The biggest strength of our study is the fact that we used a valid "gold standard" instrument to diagnose PTSD. The high cut-off used increases the specificity of the measure.

A longitudinal prospective study would be far more appropriate as it could investigate causality between attachment patterns and PTSD, but is not possible for the population that we studied. On the other hand, assessment more than 40 years after war could be an advantage, due to the delayed onset of PTSD. As we assessed lifetime PTSD 40 years after exposure has occurred, a long time has elapsed during which PTSD can develop, and, albeit possible, it is less probable that new cases will continue to occur. Furthermore, this population is increasing and is in greater need of care.

We did not assess participants' mental health, in our research, neither working models of attachment before war, and thus could not determine the direction of the associations between PTSD and attachment. Sample size was another limitation. Recall bias might have been a problem in our study, as the colonial wars ended 40 years ago. PTSD symptoms may cause a change in memories of exposure to war [69,70]. However, the way recall bias can influence the associations between war-related TEs and lifetime PTSD is difficult to ascertain in a cross-sectional study, as changes in memories can reflect dissociation or repression of events that did occur, or even the addition of false memories of events that did not occur [71]. Accordingly, childhood adversity memories can also change over such a long time of assessment after their occurrence and can also be changed by war-related trauma and lifetime PTSD. However, a recent review concluded that prospective and retrospective studies of childhood maltreatment identify different groups of mechanisms underlying psychopathology risk and that both have clinical value as risk indicators [72].

We did not study women, and thus the findings cannot be generalized for this population. The same applies to those with non-Caucasian ethnicity. Furthermore, these results cannot also be generalized for non-war-related PTSD.

5. Conclusions

Lifetime PTSD for the sample of war veterans studied is significantly associated with insecure attachment, war-related experiences, and childhood adversities. However, this study cannot conclude on the causality of the association between insecure attachment and lifetime PTSD. War-related experiences and specific childhood adversities seem to constitute significant predictors for the development of PTSD, although there is a possibility of recall bias. Severity of war exposure is associated with lifetime PTSD—independently of attachment orientations or childhood adversities. Nevertheless, the significant association of insecure attachment with lifetime PTSD assessed 40 years after war-related TEs supports the importance of attachment-focused interventions for the treatment of war veterans with lifetime PTSD.

Supplementary Materials: The following are available online at http://www.mdpi.com/2227-9032/8/4/359/s1, Supplementary Materials: War Exposure Questionnaire.

Author Contributions: Conceptualization, I.C.-V., M.S., D.C. and R.M.-C.; methodology, I.C.-V., M.S. and R.M.-C.; validation, I.C.V.; formal analysis, M.S. and I.C.-V.; investigation, I.C.-V.; resources, I.C.-V.; data curation, I.C.-V.; writing—original draft preparation, I.C.-V.; writing—review & editing, I.C.-V., M.S., D.C. and R.M.-C.; visualization, I.C.-V.; supervision, D.C.: and R.M.-C.; project administration, I.C.-V.; funding acquisition, D.C. All authors have read and agreed to the published version of the manuscript.

Funding: This work was partially supported by the Associação dos Amigos do Serviço de Endocrinologia do Hospital de São João.

Acknowledgments: We thank the Portuguese Disabled Veterans Association: Associação dos Deficientes das Forças Armadas (ADFA), for its help in selecting the sample. We also thank Sara Rocha, Cecília Aguiar, and Catarina Gomes for their assistance.

Conflicts of Interest: The authors declare no conflict of interest.

References

1. American Psychiatric Association. *Diagnostic and Statistical Manual of Mental Disorders*, 5th ed.; American Psychiatric Association: Arlington, VA, USA, 2013.
2. Breslau, N.; Kessler, R.C.; Chilcoat, H.D.; Schultz, L.R.; Davis, G.C.; Andreski, P. Trauma and posttraumatic stress disorder in the community: The 1996 Detroit area survey of trauma. *Arch. Gen. Psychiatry* **1998**, *55*, 626–632. [CrossRef]
3. DiGangi, J.A.; Gomez, D.; Mendoza, L.; Jason, L.A.; Keys, C.B.; Koenen, K.C. Pretrauma risk factors for posttraumatic stress disorder: A systematic review of the literature. *Clin. Psychol. Rev.* **2013**, *33*, 728–744. [CrossRef] [PubMed]
4. Ozer, E.J.; Best, S.R.; Lipsey, T.L.; Weiss, D.S. Predictors of posttraumatic stress disorder and symptoms in adults: A meta-analysis. *Psychol. Bull.* **2003**, *129*, 52–73. [CrossRef] [PubMed]
5. Dekel, S.; Mandl, C.; Solomon, Z. Shared and unique predictors of post-traumatic growth and distress. *J. Clin. Psychol.* **2011**, *67*, 241–252. [CrossRef] [PubMed]
6. Collins, N.L.; Ford, M.B.; Guichard, A.C.; Allard, L.M. Working models of attachment and attribution processes in intimate relationships. *Pers. Soc. Psychol. Bull.* **2006**, *32*, 201–219. [CrossRef]
7. Mikulincer, M.; Shaver, P.R. An attachment perspective on psychopathology. *World Psychiatry* **2012**, *11*, 11–15. [CrossRef]
8. Kobak, R.; Bosmans, G. Attachment and psychopathology: A dynamic model of the insecure cycle. *Curr. Opin. Psychol.* **2019**, *25*, 76–80. [CrossRef]
9. La Flair, L.N.; Bradshaw, C.P.; Mendelson, T.; Campbell, J. Intimate Partner Violence and Risk of Psychiatric Symptoms: The Moderating Role of Attachment. *J. Fam. Violence* **2015**, *30*, 567–577. [CrossRef]
10. Sandberg, D.A. Adult attachment as a predictor of posttraumatic stress and dissociation. *J. Trauma Dissociation* **2010**, *11*, 293–307. [CrossRef]
11. Lange, R.T.; Sullivan, K.A.; Scott, C. Comparison of MMPI-2 and PAI validity indicators to detect feigned depression and PTSD symptom reporting. *Psychiatry Res.* **2010**, *176*, 229–235. [CrossRef]
12. Marshall, E.M.; Frazier, P.A. Understanding posttrauma reactions within an attachment theory framework. *Curr. Opin. Psychol.* **2019**, *25*, 167–171. [CrossRef]
13. Carmassi, C.; Dell'Osso, L.; Manni, C.; Candini, V.; Dagani, J.; Iozzino, L.; Koenen, K.C.; de Girolamo, G. Frequency of trauma exposure and Post-Traumatic Stress Disorder in Italy: Analysis from the World Mental Health Survey Initiative. *J. Psychiatr. Res.* **2014**, *59*, 77–84. [CrossRef]
14. Kessler, R.C.; Sonnega, A.; Bromet, E.; Hughes, M.; Nelson, C.B. Posttraumatic stress disorder in the National Comorbidity Survey. *Arch. Gen. Psychiatry* **1995**, *52*, 1048–1060. [CrossRef]
15. Frans, O.; Rimmo, P.A.; Aberg, L.; Fredrikson, M. Trauma exposure and post-traumatic stress disorder in the general population. *Acta Psychiatr. Scand.* **2005**, *111*, 291–299. [CrossRef] [PubMed]
16. Ein-Dor, T.; Doron, G.; Solomon, Z.; Mikulincer, M.; Shaver, P.R. Together in pain: Attachment-related dyadic processes and posttraumatic stress disorder. *J. Couns. Psychol.* **2010**, *57*, 317–327. [CrossRef] [PubMed]
17. O'Connor, M.; Elklit, A. Attachment styles, traumatic events, and PTSD: A cross-sectional investigation of adult attachment and trauma. *Attach Hum. Dev.* **2008**, *10*, 59–71. [CrossRef] [PubMed]
18. Clark, A.A.; Owens, G.P. Attachment, personality characteristics, and posttraumatic stress disorder in U.S. veterans of Iraq and Afghanistan. *J. Trauma Stress* **2012**, *25*, 657–664. [CrossRef]
19. Currier, J.M.; Holland, J.M.; Allen, D. Attachment and mental health symptoms among U.S. Afghanistan and Iraq veterans seeking health care services. *J. Trauma Stress* **2012**, *25*, 633–640. [CrossRef]
20. Franz, C.E.; Lyons, M.J.; Spoon, K.M.; Hauger, R.L.; Jacobson, K.C.; Lohr, J.B.; McKenzie, R.; Panizzon, M.S.; Thompson, W.K.; Tsuang, M.T.; et al. Post-traumatic stress symptoms and adult attachment: A 24-year longitudinal study. *Am. J. Geriatr. Psychiatry* **2014**, *22*, 1603–1612. [CrossRef]
21. Solomon, Z.; Dekel, R.; Mikulincer, M. Complex trauma of war captivity: A prospective study of attachment and post-traumatic stress disorder. *Psychol. Med.* **2008**, *38*, 1427–1434. [CrossRef]

22. Weinfield, N.S.; Sroufe, L.A.; Egeland, B. Attachment from infancy to early adulthood in a high-risk sample: Continuity, discontinuity, and their correlates. *Child. Dev.* **2000**, *71*, 695–702. [CrossRef] [PubMed]
23. van Zuiden, M.; Geuze, E.; Willemen, H.L.; Vermetten, E.; Maas, M.; Amarouchi, K.; Kavelaars, A.; Heijnen, C.J. Glucocorticoid receptor pathway components predict posttraumatic stress disorder symptom development: A prospective study. *Biol. Psychiatry* **2012**, *71*, 309–316. [CrossRef] [PubMed]
24. Muller, R.T.; Sicoli, L.A.; Lemieux, K.E. Relationship between attachment style and posttraumatic stress symptomatology among adults who report the experience of childhood abuse. *J. Trauma Stress* **2000**, *13*, 321–332. [CrossRef] [PubMed]
25. Muller, R.T.; Thornback, K.; Bedi, R. Attachment as a Mediator between Childhood Maltreatment and Adult Symptomatology. *J. Fam. Violence* **2012**, *27*, 243–255. [CrossRef]
26. LeardMann, C.A.; Smith, B.; Ryan, M.A. Do adverse childhood experiences increase the risk of postdeployment posttraumatic stress disorder in US Marines? *BMC Public Health* **2010**, *10*, 437. [CrossRef]
27. Kolassa, I.T.; Kolassa, S.; Ertl, V.; Papassotiropoulos, A.; De Quervain, D.J. The risk of posttraumatic stress disorder after trauma depends on traumatic load and the catechol-o-methyltransferase Val(158)Met polymorphism. *Biol. Psychiatry* **2010**, *67*, 304–308. [CrossRef]
28. Berntsen, D.; Johannessen, K.B.; Thomsen, Y.D.; Bertelsen, M.; Hoyle, R.H.; Rubin, D.C. Peace and war: Trajectories of posttraumatic stress disorder symptoms before, during, and after military deployment in Afghanistan. *Psychol. Sci.* **2012**, *23*, 1557–1565. [CrossRef]
29. Polusny, M.A.; Erbes, C.R.; Murdoch, M.; Arbisi, P.A.; Thuras, P.; Rath, M.B. Prospective risk factors for new-onset post-traumatic stress disorder in National Guard soldiers deployed to Iraq. *Psychol. Med.* **2011**, *41*, 687–698. [CrossRef]
30. Rona, R.J.; Hooper, R.; Jones, M.; Iversen, A.C.; Hull, L.; Murphy, D.; Hotopf, M.; Wessely, S. The contribution of prior psychological symptoms and combat exposure to post Iraq deployment mental health in the UK military. *J. Trauma Stress* **2009**, *22*, 11–19. [CrossRef]
31. Litz, B.T.; Stein, N.; Delaney, E.; Lebowitz, L.; Nash, W.P.; Silva, C.; Maguen, S. Moral injury and moral repair in war veterans: A preliminary model and intervention strategy. *Clin. Psychol. Rev.* **2009**, *29*, 695–706. [CrossRef]
32. Maia, A.; McIntyre, T.; Pereira, M.G.; Ribeiro, E. War exposure and post-traumatic stress as predictors of Portuguese colonial war veterans' physical health. *Anxiety Stress Coping* **2011**, *24*, 309–325. [CrossRef] [PubMed]
33. Port, C.L.; Engdahl, B.; Frazier, P. A longitudinal and retrospective study of PTSD among older prisoners of war. *Am. J. Psychiatry* **2001**, *158*, 1474–1479. [CrossRef] [PubMed]
34. Steenkamp, M.M.; Litz, B.T.; Hoge, C.W.; Marmar, C.R. Psychotherapy for Military-Related PTSD: A Review of Randomized Clinical Trials. *JAMA* **2015**, *314*, 489–500. [CrossRef]
35. Castro-Vale, I.; Severo, M.; Carvalho, D.; Mota-Cardoso, R. Intergenerational transmission of war-related trauma assessed 40 years after exposure. *Ann. Gen. Psychiatry* **2019**, *18*, 14. [CrossRef]
36. American Psychiatric Association. *Diagnostic and Statistical Manual of Mental Disorders*, 4th ed.; Text Revision; American Psychiatric Association: Washington, DC, USA, 2000.
37. Graffar, M. Une methode de classification sociales d'echantillons de population. *Courrier* **1956**, *6*, 445–459. (In French)
38. Costa, A.M.B.; Leitão, F.R.; Santos, J.; Pinto, J.V.; Fino, M.N. Formulários utilizados na caracterização do aluno no seu contexto familiar, escolar e social e na elaboração do programa educativo. In *Currículos Funcionais*; Instituto de Inovação Educacional: Lisboa, Portugal, 1996; Volume 2, pp. 11–60. (In Portuguese)
39. Blake, D.D.; Weathers, F.W.; Nagy, L.M.; Kaloupek, D.G.; Gusman, F.D.; Charney, D.S.; Keane, T.M. The development of a Clinician-Administered PTSD Scale. *J. Trauma Stress* **1995**, *8*, 75–90. [CrossRef] [PubMed]
40. Blake, D.D.; Weathers, F.; Nagy, L.M.; Kaloupek, D.G.; Klauminzer, G.; Charney, D.; Keane, T. A clinician rating scale for assessing current and lifetime PTSD: The CAPS-1. *Behav. Ther.* **1990**, *13*, 187–188.
41. First, M.B.; Spitzer, R.L.; Gibbon, M.; Williams, J.B.W. *Structured Clinical Interview for DSM-IV Axis I Disorders, Clinician Version (SCID-CV)*; American Psychiatric Press, Inc.: Washington, DC, USA, 1996.
42. Bernstein, D.P.; Stein, J.A.; Newcomb, M.D.; Walker, E.; Pogge, D.; Ahluvalia, T.; Stokes, J.; Handelsman, L.; Medrano, M.; Desmond, D.; et al. Development and validation of a brief screening version of the Childhood Trauma Questionnaire. *Child Abus. Negl.* **2003**, *27*, 169–190. [CrossRef]

43. Dias, A.; Sales, L.; Carvalho, A.; Castro Vale, I.; Kleber, R.; Mota Cardoso, R. Estudo de propriedades psicométricas do Questionário de Trauma de Infância—Versão breve numa amostra portuguesa não clínica. *Lab. Psicol.* **2014**, *11*, 103–120. (In Portuguese) [CrossRef]
44. Canavarro, M.C.; Dias, P.; Lima, V. A avaliação da vinculação do adulto: Uma revisão crítica a propósito da aplicação da Adult Attachment Scale-R (AAS-R) na população portuguesa. *Psicologia* **2006**, *20*, 155–187. (In Portuguese) [CrossRef]
45. Collins, N.L. Working models of attachment: Implications for explanation, emotion and behavior. *J. Pers. Soc. Psychol.* **1996**, *71*, 810–832. [CrossRef] [PubMed]
46. Bartholomew, K. Avoidance of Intimacy: An Attachment Perspective. *J. Soc. Pers. Relatsh.* **1990**, *7*, 147–178. [CrossRef]
47. Fraley, R.C.; Roisman, G.I. The development of adult attachment styles: Four lessons. *Curr. Opin. Psychol.* **2019**, *25*, 26–30. [CrossRef] [PubMed]
48. Trappler, B.; Braunstein, J.W.; Moskowitz, G.; Friedman, S. Holocaust survivors in a primary care setting: Fifty years later. *Psychol. Rep.* **2002**, *91*, 545–552. [CrossRef] [PubMed]
49. Woodhouse, S.; Ayers, S.; Field, A.P. The relationship between adult attachment style and post-traumatic stress symptoms: A meta-analysis. *J. Anxiety Disord.* **2015**, *35*, 103–117. [CrossRef]
50. Ortigo, K.M.; Westen, D.; Defife, J.A.; Bradley, B. Attachment, social cognition, and posttraumatic stress symptoms in a traumatized, urban population: Evidence for the mediating role of object relations. *J. Trauma Stress* **2013**, *26*, 361–368. [CrossRef]
51. Armour, C.; Elklit, A.; Shevlin, M. Attachment typologies and posttraumatic stress disorder (PTSD), depression and anxiety: A latent profile analysis approach. *Eur. J. Psychotraumatol.* **2011**, *2*, 6018. [CrossRef]
52. Bateman, A.W.; Ryle, A.; Fonagy, P.; Kerr, I.B. Psychotherapy for borderline personality disorder: Mentalization based therapy and cognitive analytic therapy compared. *Int. Rev. Psychiatry* **2007**, *19*, 51–62. [CrossRef]
53. Keenan, M.J.; Lumley, V.A.; Schneider, R.B. A group therapy approach to treating combat posttraumatic stress disorder: Interpersonal reconnection through letter writing. *Psychotherapy* **2014**, *51*, 546–554. [CrossRef]
54. Slade, A.; Holmes, J. Attachment and psychotherapy. *Curr. Opin. Psychol.* **2019**, *25*, 152–156. [CrossRef]
55. Stovall-McClough, K.C.; Cloitre, M. Reorganization of unresolved childhood traumatic memories following exposure therapy. *Ann. N. Y. Acad. Sci.* **2003**, *1008*, 297–299. [CrossRef] [PubMed]
56. Thorp, S.R.; Glassman, L.H.; Wells, S.Y.; Walter, K.H.; Gebhardt, H.; Twamley, E.; Golshan, S.; Pittman, J.; Penski, K.; Allard, C.; et al. A randomized controlled trial of prolonged exposure therapy versus relaxation training for older veterans with military-related PTSD. *J. Anxiety Disord.* **2019**, *64*, 45–54. [CrossRef] [PubMed]
57. Dimaggio, G. To expose or not to expose? The integrative therapist and posttraumatic stress disorder. *J. Psychother. Integr.* **2019**, *29*, 1–5. [CrossRef]
58. Kelly, A.; Garland, E.L. Trauma-informed mindfulness-based stress reduction for female survivors of interpersonal violence: Results from a stage I RCT. *J. Clin. Psychol.* **2016**, *72*, 311–328. [CrossRef] [PubMed]
59. Steelman, B. Attachment-based therapy for elder suffering PTSD symptoms: A narrative of modeling efficacy for improved outcomes. *Perspect. Psychiatr. Care* **2019**, *55*, 72–74. [CrossRef] [PubMed]
60. Forbes, D.; Parslow, R.; Fletcher, S.; McHugh, T.; Creamer, M. Attachment style in the prediction of recovery following group treatment of combat veterans with post-traumatic stress disorder. *J. Nerv. Ment. Dis.* **2010**, *198*, 881–884. [CrossRef] [PubMed]
61. Dias, A.; Sales, L.; Cardoso, R.M.; Kleber, R. Childhood maltreatment in adult offspring of Portuguese war veterans with and without PTSD. *Eur. J. Psychotraumatol.* **2014**, *5*, 20198. [CrossRef]
62. van Zuiden, M.; Geuze, E.; Willemen, H.L.; Vermetten, E.; Maas, M.; Heijnen, C.J.; Kavelaars, A. Pre-existing high glucocorticoid receptor number predicting development of posttraumatic stress symptoms after military deployment. *Am. J. Psychiatry* **2011**, *168*, 89–96. [CrossRef]
63. Brewin, C.R.; Andrews, B.; Valentine, J.D. Meta-analysis of risk factors for posttraumatic stress disorder in trauma-exposed adults. *J. Consult. Clin. Psychol.* **2000**, *68*, 748–766. [CrossRef]
64. Breslau, N.; Peterson, E.L. Assaultive violence and the risk of posttraumatic stress disorder following a subsequent trauma. *Behav. Res. Ther.* **2010**, *48*, 1063–1066. [CrossRef]
65. Breslau, N.; Peterson, E.L.; Schultz, L.R. A second look at prior trauma and the posttraumatic stress disorder effects of subsequent trauma: A prospective epidemiological study. *Arch. Gen. Psychiatry* **2008**, *65*, 431–437. [CrossRef] [PubMed]

66. Bremner, J.D.; Southwick, S.M.; Johnson, D.R.; Yehuda, R.; Charney, D.S. Childhood physical abuse and combat-related posttraumatic stress disorder in Vietnam veterans. *Am. J. Psychiatry* **1993**, *150*, 235–239. [CrossRef] [PubMed]
67. Dunmore, E.; Clark, D.M.; Ehlers, A. Cognitive factors involved in the onset and maintenance of posttraumatic stress disorder (PTSD) after physical or sexual assault. *Behav. Res. Ther.* **1999**, *37*, 809–829. [CrossRef]
68. Fear, N.T.; Jones, M.; Murphy, D.; Hull, L.; Iversen, A.C.; Coker, B.; Machell, L.; Sundin, J.; Woodhead, C.; Jones, N.; et al. What are the consequences of deployment to Iraq and Afghanistan on the mental health of the UK armed forces? A cohort study. *Lancet* **2010**, *375*, 1783–1797. [CrossRef]
69. Southwick, S.M.; Morgan, C.A., III; Nicolaou, A.L.; Charney, D.S. Consistency of memory for combat-related traumatic events in veterans of Operation Desert Storm. *Am. J. Psychiatry* **1997**, *154*, 173–177. [CrossRef]
70. Wessely, S.; Unwin, C.; Hotopf, M.; Hull, L.; Ismail, K.; Nicolaou, V.; David, A. Stability of recall of military hazards over time. Evidence from the Persian Gulf War of 1991. *Br. J. Psychiatry* **2003**, *183*, 314–322. [CrossRef]
71. Spiegel, D. Consistency of memory among veterans of Operation Desert Storm. *Am. J. Psychiatry* **1998**, *155*, 1301. [CrossRef]
72. Syed Sheriff, R.; Van Hooff, M.; Malhi, G.S.; Grace, B.; McFarlane, A. Childhood determinants of past-year anxiety and depression in recently transitioned military personnel. *J. Affect. Disord.* **2020**, *274*, 59–66. [CrossRef]

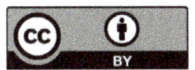

© 2020 by the authors. Licensee MDPI, Basel, Switzerland. This article is an open access article distributed under the terms and conditions of the Creative Commons Attribution (CC BY) license (http://creativecommons.org/licenses/by/4.0/).

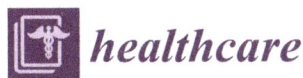

Article

A Qualitative Case Study on Influencing Factors of Parents' Child Abuse of North Korean Refugees in South Korea

Wonjung Ryu and Hyerin Yang *

The Center for Social Welfare Research, Yonsei University, Seoul 03722, Korea; wjryu514@gmail.com
* Correspondence: rinyang0103@gmail.com; Tel.: +82-10-3443-8712

Received: 2 December 2020; Accepted: 30 December 2020; Published: 5 January 2021

Abstract: The purpose of this study is to investigate the influencing factors of parental child abuse by North Korean refugees who are living in South Korea. In-depth interviews were conducted with five parents who escaped from North Korea. The study identified three categories of factors impacting child abuse: the weakening of family functions from past experiences before and after defection, the stress of adapting to the culture of an unfamiliar society, and low parenting self-efficacy. North Korean parents suffered from emotional and functional crises from past traumatic events and, at the same time, experienced additional acculturative stress as a "minority" after entering South Korea, even as they continued to deal with Maternal Parenting Stress. These complex factors have been shown to lead to child abuse in migrant societies. This study contemplated the context of child abuse through specific examples. The results could provide thoughtful insights into child abuse among migrants and refugee parents, and provide evidence-based intervention plans for its prevention.

Keywords: North Korean refugees; child abuse; acculturative stress; parenting self-efficacy; qualitative case study

1. Introduction

North Korea's communist regime has been committing human rights violations throughout its three-generation-long reign of terror. Even at this moment, many North Koreans are in various kinds of anti-human-rights situations, enduring violence, torture, hunger, and social control. For this reason, many try to escape every year. South Korean society refers to those who have escaped from North Korea as 'North Korean refugees' ('NK refugees').

The number of NK refugees who have defected from the North and settled in the South is now at about 37,000 [1]. The entry of NK refugees to South Korea has gradually increased since the 1990's when the severe economic crisis began in North Korea, with more than 1000 NK refugees still entering South Korea every year [1] (p. 1). As the number of NK refugees has increased over the past two decades, a new type of family, termed a "North Korean family" (an 'NK family') has been created in South Korea. While the correct figures have not been aggregated recently, the pattern of escaping from North Korea with 'family units' has been increasing. And the fact that 77.3% of NK refugees in South Korea in their 40's or younger [1] (p. 1), thus in their childbearing years, implies that NK families could gradually become a meaningful family type in South Korean society. It is easy to erroneously believe that all members of North Korean refugee families are actually from North Korea, but by looking deeper into the families, it becomes clear that their countries of origin vary, including people from North Korea, China, and South Korea, due to human trafficking, separation, reunion, and remarriage in the process of defection. This means that many NK families have low family bonds and cohesion, which results in frequent family conflicts or domestic violence.

In fact, according to a recent survey, 49% of NK refugees have physically abused their children, while 57.7% of them have ever committed emotional abuse [2]. This figure is about three times higher than the ratio of South Korean parents' abuse identified in the same survey. This clearly shows NK refugee vulnerability around the issue of child abuse.

The problem of child abuse is serious not only among NK refugees' families but also in other refugee families in Western society. Previous research has shown that child abuse in refugee families is more prevalent than among ordinary immigrant families, and they pointed out that it can occur in different patterns [3,4].

A multitude of services and interventions are being developed as social concerns over refugee family abuse gradually increase, but NK refugees have another different character compared to other refugees. Therefore, understanding these families' specific nature and environments is very important to solve the problem of child abuse in NK refugees' families. Unlike other refugees, NK refugees experienced fear from the reign of terror in North Korea, and they have been forced into particular actions and beliefs in a 'completely controlled society' for the past 70 years. Examples include forcing a belief that denies capitalism or providing socialist education based on loyalty to the leader. After entering South Korea, they face additional pressures, having to adapt quickly to a new society, experiencing a lot of stress due to job insecurity, economic difficulties, a lack of support, discrimination, and exclusion from South Korean society. They are also unstable in their roles as parents or have low confidence in their parenting abilities [5]. Such transitional experiences and processes make the risk of child abuse more higher.

The South Korean government and many NK refugee support organizations are actively looking for social services and interventions to prevent child abuse overall, but they currently lack a concrete approach to 'NK families.' The interventions for preventing child abuse should be implemented based on an understanding of the specific situations NK refugees' families face because this is a good way to increase the effectiveness of prevention strategies and mitigate the recurrence of abuse. Therefore, this study, based on the qualitative interviews with NK refugee parents, identifies specific reasons why child abuse occurs within their family context, and ultimately seeks to examine measures that could prevent child abuse.

1.1. Characteristics of NK Refugee Families Living in South Korea

In order to understand the child abuse behaviors of NK refugees, one must first consider the characteristics of NK refugees' families and the main characteristics of their distinctive environment.

First, NK refugees experience serious trauma during their defection. There are three main routes of defection to enter South Korea: ① via China; ② via East Asian countries through China; or ③ via Mongolia through China. Throughout the ordeal, a large number of NK refugees confront life-and-death situations. According to a previous study, 96.5% of NK refugees endured more than one traumatic event [6]. The study found that they experienced incidents repeatedly, which rarely happens to ordinary people in their lifetime [7], with trials encompassing food shortages, labor camp imprisonment, torture and beatings, human trafficking, and having to avoid arrest by the secret police. Unfortunately, they also experienced many traumatic events after arriving in South Korea because the social, economic, and cultural environments between the two countries have diverged since their division more than half a century ago. As the traditional culture in which these North Koreans had lived with is, for the most part, not accepted by South Korean society, they repeatedly face social discrimination and stigma in their daily lives caused by acculturative stress [8,9].

> *"I finally got a chance to meet my kid after four years, but he didn't want to talk to me for three months. I tried to have a conversation but he almost refused ... [skip] He kept behaving in that way, which made me stop trying to put effort into him."* [Participant E]

3.1.2. Emotional Disorders of Parents Caused by Traumatic Events

Most of the participants in the study experienced trauma in the process of escaping. One of them witnessed their daughter being shot to death during the escape; another was tortured at an NK detention facility after being arrested. Other participants also experienced a serious life crisis during that time. They experienced severe after-effects such as depression, isolation, and PTSD from past experiences, and it directly affected their parenting. Participant B confessed that she struggled with the trauma and couldn't do anything for three months, which eventually made her abuse her child badly. Participant D said that after the dangerous defection, she became aggressive and her sense of victimization became very severe. This emotional condition had a negative impact on child-rearing, with her becoming sensitive to the child's words and behaviors, and becoming a person who easily got mad at her child's tiny mistakes.

> *"The previous memories repeatedly coming to my mind, I couldn't do well in my daily life for several months. I felt depressed, sad, lonely ... and I didn't even want to see my child playing. So I sometimes hurt him."* [Participant B]

> *"Since past trauma experiences, I've become angry and impulsive. So I was more likely to be mad at my kid, hurting him by talking in a bad way."* [Participant D]

3.2. Acculturative Stress in South Korean Society

3.2.1. Stress Expression and Transfer during the Child-Rearing Process

NK refugee parents were found to be very stressed by South Korean society. They were filled with depression and fury by the discrimination, exclusion, and tendency to recognize them as 'strangers' that they faced in South Korean society. This situation made it difficult for them to think normally and exacerbated even small problems in the child-rearing process. Participant E, whose defection motivation was for her 'children's future,' transferred the stress and the related emotions that occurred during the adaptation process onto her children. Sometimes she threatened to send them back to China. In this way, the children became the object of their parents' anger. Participant C said that excessive stress brought about in the process of adapting caused a sense of helplessness in her life, which led to the neglect of her children.

> *"It's not easy to live in South Korea being treated as a 'stranger' and I ended up getting angry at my child. Thinking of it, it was not a big deal ... (skip) but I said a lot of acrimonious things to him. When I was angry, I even told him that I'll send him back to China, and one day he said it really hurt him."* [Participant E]

> *"The pressures ... I gave all to my child. Even if my child was hungry, I left him alone."* [Participant C]

In the case of participant A, the more stressed she felt in South Korean society, the more obsessed she was with her child's performance and success, recognizing 'children' as the only factor to get out of the stressful reality. This led to excessive interference and control of her children's behavior, and to her raising them under strict discipline and with corporal punishment.

> *"Well, I thought living here, in South Korea, after all the tough times, would be worth it only when my kid succeeds in his career. So, I think I've become more obsessed with him."* [Participant A]

3.2.2. Conflicts Due to Differences in Adaptation Levels between Parents and Children

NK refugee children have turned out to be relatively less stressed and faster at adapting to life in South Korea than their parents. These differences in adaptation level are found to cause differences in values between parents and children, and to eventually deepen the conflicts between parents and children. In the case of participant C, her children, who adapted quickly to South Korea, had a high level of comprehension in democracy, human rights, and equal family culture. And when facing conflicts, parents felt ignored or challenged to exert parental authority over their children who claim these values. These feelings have led parents to more strict discipline and corporal punishment than ever. Some North Korean parents also thought that abuse had the effect of weakening their children's rebellious behavior, which led them to stick to abusive parenting or to gradually increase the level of their abuse.

> *"They've already changed quickly after entering South Korea. One day, my child talked back to me about equality and human rights, and I don't now why . . . but I felt unpleasant, so I scolded him."* [Participant C]

> *"As my child has grown up, I thought that my authority had become ignored and challenged by him. Sometimes I hurt him physically as I thought he'd keep ignoring me if I don't scold him."* [Participant B]

3.3. Decrease in Parenting Efficacy

3.3.1. Confusion in the Role of Parents before and after Migration

NK refugees experienced confusion in their parenting roles in the process of migrating to a new society, and they felt frustration around bringing up their kids. According to participant D, whenever their parenting behaviors learned in North Korea were considered a bad parenting style in South Korean society, they felt confused about their role as parents. Excessive interference and criticism form South Korean society reduced their confidence in parenting further. This low parenting efficacy has caused child abuse.

> *"In some cases, the parenting beliefs that I have had from North Korea was considered a child abuse act in South Korean society. It was confusing, so I tried to change the way of raising my kids many times, but it didn't help but just confused my kids too."* [Participant D]

3.3.2. Lack of Parenting Information

The shortage of parenting information was a common characteristic among NK refugee parents. Since there are no parenting education programs in North Korea, NK refugee parents enter into the South without knowledge relating to parenting. South Korea currently has a variety of parental education programs, but lacks customized parenting education programs for NK refugees. Aside from this, it is very difficult for those who have to engage in irregular economic activities to participate in education programs. The NK refugee parents also lack social support resources, so they do not have supporters to turn to and ask for help when raising children is difficult. Thus, they gradually lose confidence in their role as parents. The problem is that in such cases, they tend to choose a corporal punishment-oriented parenting style, which is familiar to them from their North Korean culture.

> *"I heard that there are many parenting education programs in South Korea, but it doesn't really help us as it is more important for us to make money than learning from the program. So . . . I raise my child by how I learned in North Korea."* [Participant A]

In sum, NK refugee parents experience emotional crises and stress in the process of defection, which weakens the functionality of the family or individual. These risk factors affect their parenting style. The three meta-categories identified in this study as single factors directly affect the way children are raised and are associated with abusive behavior. This study confirmed that the factors are interrelated and induce child abuse. Moreover, the absence of protective factors, such as support resources and parenting information in South Korean society were revealed to make their abusive behavior tendencies more serious.

4. Discussion

This study has important academic value in that it has identified the factors of NK refugees' child abuse behaviors within the specific context of migration. The results of this study show that, from their experiences during the process of defection, NK refugees have weakened their personal and family functions, which negatively affects their attachment and family bonding, thereby indirectly increasing the risk of abuse. Specifically, North Korean parents who experienced traumatic events in the past have suffered from severe after-effects such as depression and PTSD, which were identified as having a direct impact on parenting style. The results are consistent with studies by Chan [29] and Harrington & Dubowitz [30], who demonstrated a relationship between parental emotional problems and child abuse. Today, services for migrant and refugee families, including NK refugees, are mainly focused on economic support [31], but this study shows that emotional recovery services such as psychological treatment and counseling for past experiences and trauma are equally important.

This study determined that stress arising from the adaptation of NK refugee parents has a great effect on child abuse. This is similar to studies on immigration and refugees of Hispanic and Vietnamese communities [21,22] (p. 3). The results of this study show that the stress experienced by NK refugees during migration caused psychological problems like depression, helplessness, and aggression, which led to negative attitudes in parenting.

Moreover, NK refugee parents with patriarchal attitudes were concerned about losing their authority over their children who were quicker to adapt, which led to stricter discipline and corporal punishment. These results suggest that they need direct and active interventions such as anger control programs, stress relief programs, and cognitive-behavioral programs for NK refugee parents. In addition, providing self-help clubs and mentoring services with their South Korean neighbors could eliminate the sense of isolation and alienation, which, in turn, would then allow them to adapt better in South Korean society.

Finally, NK refugee parents showed low parenting efficacy due to confusion in their parenting style and lack of parenting information, and the low parenting efficacy was related to child abuse. This is consistent with studies by [32–34] Luster & Kain, Shin and Ahn, which identified that the lower the parenting efficacy, the more they were inclined to emphasize discipline and coercive parenting. The result of this study is similar to [35] Gross et al.'s study, in that the higher the efficacy of parenting, the more positive the parenting tended to be. Along with confusion about parenting, they tended to choose a parenting pattern that they learned in North Korea, a method that focused on physical punishment. This phenomenon is more often found in parents who have migrated from countries with a patriarchal culture and, as expected, it is also seen in parents of North Korean refugee families. So, in light of the results of this study, thinking seriously about their parenting role is a necessity. In other words, it seems that they need customized parenting education programs that can improve their efficacy.

The educational content should be focused on changing misunderstandings about the parenting role and disseminating useful parenting knowledge. Considering that they are NK refugees who lack the time to participate in educational programs due to low wages and job insecurity, other ways, such as offering incentives or providing online education, could also be helpful.

5. Limitations

This study lacked diversity among the subjects. The study was conducted with only those participants who expressed their willingness to participate, so parents who engage in unstable employment situations were excluded. Therefore, follow-up research should try to include various NK participants, including single parents and young parents who may have more difficulty raising their children. In addition, in-depth interviews were difficult in this study. In order to understand the details, additional questions such as the background of their defection, and information about family members remaining in the North are sometimes required, but there is a limitation as questions were difficult, considering the sensitivity of the questions and the participants' emotions. In addition, if it was determined that there was an expected risk of information exposure, even if the information was voluntarily stated by participants, the issue was not actively addressed in this study.

6. Conclusions

This qualitative research found that the issue of child abuse by NK refugees' parents arises in a specific context of migration. This is similar to studies of migrant and refugee families abroad. We suggest that service providers should consider the culture and experience of both the entry country and migrant country when intervening in their problem. Similarly, child abuse prevention services previously designed for non-refugee families present many limitations to NK refugee families. Therefore, the government, local governments, and related organizations should develop child abuse prevention programs that consider the specific needs of NK refugees.

Previous results show that child abuse is more likely to be caused by personal, emotional, cognitive, and environmental factors that are interrelated and, influencing each other, rather than being caused by a single factor. This conversely suggests that utilizing the 'virtuous circle of resources' for the prevention of abuse is possible. In other words, intervention in some factors may affect others since the factors are linked together. Therefore, it is necessary to consider the structural relationship and the size of influence of each risk factor when balancing realistic problems as they arise in practice, such as when prioritizing the service supply is necessary due to limited resources.

In addition, in this study, the mechanism of occurrence of abuse by case was found to be very specific, diverse, and contextual. Therefore, the intervention for preventing child abuse is expected to be more effective if service providers add to their efforts to closely assess the individual circumstances and context they are in.

Author Contributions: W.R. and H.Y. contributed equally to all aspects of the research reported in this paper. All authors have read and agreed to the published version of the manuscript.

Funding: This research received no external funding.

Institutional Review Board Statement: The study was conducted according to the guidelines of the Declaration of Helsinki, and approved by the Ethics Committee of Yonsei University (protocol code: 7001988-201810-HR-408-04, date of approval: 29 June 2018).

Informed Consent Statement: Informed consent was obtained from all subjects involved in the study.

Data Availability Statement: The data presented in this study are available on request from the corresponding author. The data are not publicly available due to Participant's personal information.

Conflicts of Interest: The authors declare no potential conflicts of interest with respect to the research, authorship and/or publication of this article.

References

1. Korea National Statistical Office. *Status of NK Refugees Living in South Korea*; Korea National Statistical Office: Daejon, Korea, 2020.
2. Ministry of Gender Equality and Family. *2010 Korean National Survey on Domestic Violence*; Ministry of Gender Equality and Family: Seoul, Korea, 2010.
3. LeBrun, A.; Hassan, G.; Boivin, M.; Fraser, S.L.; Dufour, S.; Lavergne, C. Review of child maltreatment in immigrant and refugee families. *Can. J. Public Health* **2015**, *106*, eS45–eS56. [CrossRef] [PubMed]
4. Hassan, G.; Thombs, B.D.; Rousseau, C.; Kirmayer, L.J.; Feightner, J.; Ueffing, E.; Pottie, K. Child Maltreatment: Evidence Review for Newly Arriving Immigrants and Refugees. *Can. Med. Assoc. J.* **2011**, *183*, 1–15.
5. Park, S.; An, S. A Study on the Variables Affecting Parenting Efficacy of North Korean Refugee Mothers: With a Focus on Marital Satisfaction, Social Support, and Acculturation. *Korean J. Child. Stud.* **2014**, *35*, 103–122. [CrossRef]
6. Kim, T.G.; Jung, E.E. Relationship between time after Traumatic experience and Posttraumatic Growth of North Korean defectors. *Korean J. Psychol.* **2014**, *1*, 257.
7. Yang, H.R. A Study of Traumatic Event Experiences and Post-Traumatic Growth (PTG) among NK Adolescent Refugees in South Korea. Master's Thesis, Yonsei University, Seoul, South Korea, 1 August 2018.
8. Jo, Y.A. The Effect of Perceived discrimination on Psychological distress among North Korean refugees. *Korea J. Couns.* **2011**, *12*, 1–19.
9. Lee, B.M. A Qualitative Study on the Process of Adaptation of North Korean Parents in South Korean Society. *J. Korean Counc. Child. Rights* **2005**, *9*, 691–726.
10. Kim, H. The Family Characteristics and Uneven Changes in North Korea. *Korea J. Fam. Cult.* **2017**, *29*, 67–104.
11. Lee, H. The Identity Change Process of Women Defectors of North Korea through Emigrant Experiences. *J. Women Stud.* **2011**, *21*, 173–211.
12. Park, H.; Kim, Y.; Park, H. Grounded Theory Approach to Transition Process of Parenting Experience among Mothers Defecting from North Korean. *Child Health Nurs. Res.* **2011**, *17*, 48–57. [CrossRef]
13. Lee, I.S.; Park, H.R.; Park, H.J.; Park, Y.H. Relationships between parenting behavior, parenting efficacy, adaptation stress and post traumatic stress disorder among mothers who defected from North Korean. *Child Health Nurs. Res.* **2010**, *16*, 360–368. [CrossRef]
14. Berry, J.W. Acculturation. In *Handbook of Socialization: Theory and Research*; Gusec, J.E., Hastings, P.D., Eds.; Guilford Press: New York, NY, USA, 2007; pp. 543–558.
15. Martins, V.; Reid, D. New-immigrant women in urban Canada: Insights into occupation and sociocultural context. *Occup. Ther. Int.* **2007**, *14*, 203–220. [CrossRef] [PubMed]
16. Weerasinghe, W.; Mitchell, T. Connection between the meaning of health and interaction with health professionals: Caring for immigrant women. *Health Care Women Int.* **2007**, *28*, 309–328. [CrossRef] [PubMed]
17. Ahn, J.Y.; Park, S.Y. The effects of maternal parental beliefs, efficacy and stress on mother's parenting behaviors. *J. Korean Home Econ. Assoc.* **2002**, *40*, 53–68.
18. Lundahl, B.W.; Nimer, J.; Parsons, B. Preventing child abuse: A meta-analysis of parent training programs. *Res. Soc. Work Pract.* **2006**, *16*, 251–262. [CrossRef]
19. Cicchetti, D.; Rogosch, F.A.; Toth, S.L. The efficacy of toddler-parent psychotherapy for fostering cognitive development in offspring of depressed mothers. *J. Abnorm. Child Psychol.* **2000**, *28*, 135–148. [CrossRef]
20. Segal, U.A.; Mayadas, N.S. Assessment of issues facing immigrant and refugee families. *Child Welf.* **2005**, *84*, 563–583.
21. Zayas, L.H. Childrearing, social stress, and child abuse: Clinical considerations with Hispanic families. *J. Soc. Distress Homeless* **1992**, *1*, 291–309. [CrossRef]
22. Rhee, S.; Chang, J.; Berthold, S.M.; Mar, G. Child maltreatment among immigrant Vietnamese families: Characteristics and implications for practice. *Child Adolesc. Soc. Work J.* **2012**, *29*, 85–101. [CrossRef]
23. Coleman, P.K.; Karraker, K.H. Parenting self-efficacy among mothers of school-age children: Conceptualization, measurement, and correlates. *Fam. Relat.* **2000**, *49*, 13–24. [CrossRef]

24. Gondoli, D.M.; Silverberg, S.B. Maternal emotional distress and diminished responsiveness: The mediating role of parenting efficacy and parental perspective taking. *Dev. Psychol.* **1997**, *33*, 861–868. [CrossRef]
25. Teti, D.M.; Gelfand, D.M. Behavioral competence among mothers of infants in the first year: The mediational role of maternal self-efficacy. *Child Dev.* **1991**, *62*, 918–929. [CrossRef] [PubMed]
26. Coleman, P.K.; Karraker, K.H. Self-efficacy and parenting quality: Findings and future applications. *Dev. Rev.* **1998**, *18*, 47–85. [CrossRef]
27. Dumka, L.E.; Stoerzinger, H.D.; Jackson, K.M.; Roosa, M.W. Examination of the cross-cultural and cross-language equivalence of the parenting self-agency measure. *Fam. Relat.* **1996**, *45*, 216–222. [CrossRef]
28. Stake, R.E. *The Art of Case Study Research*; Sage Publications: New York, NY, USA, 1995.
29. Chan, Y.C. Parenting stress and social support of mothers who physically abuse their children in Hong Kong. *Child. Abus. Negl.* **1994**, *18*, 261–269. [CrossRef]
30. Harrington, D.; Dubowitz, H. Preventing child maltreatment. In *Family Violence: Prevention and Treatment*, 2nd ed.; Hampton, R.L., Ed.; Sage Publications: New York, NY, USA, 1999.
31. Yang, H.; Ryu, W. A Study of Post-traumatic Growth (PTG) among North Korean Adolescent Refugees in South Korea: Classifying latent profiles in growth and testing the effects of determinants. *Korean J. Adolesc. Welf.* **2020**, *22*, 139–167. [CrossRef]
32. Luster, T.; Kain, E.L. The relation between family context and perceptions of parental efficacy. *Early Child Dev. Care* **1987**, *29*, 301–311. [CrossRef]
33. Sin, S.J. Effects of Stress, Social Support and Efficacy on Mothers' Parenting Behaviors. *Korean J. Child Stud.* **1998**, *19*, 27–42.
34. Ahn, J.Y. The Effects of Maternal Parental Beliefs, Efficacy and Stress on Mother's Parenting Behaviors. Master's Thesis, Ehwa University, Seoul, South Korea, 31 January 2001.
35. Gross, D.; Conrad, B.; Fogg, L.; Wothke, W. A longitudinal model of maternal self-efficacy, depression, and difficult temperament during toddlerhood. *Res. Nurs. Health* **1994**, *17*, 207–215. [CrossRef]

Publisher's Note: MDPI stays neutral with regard to jurisdictional claims in published maps and institutional affiliations.

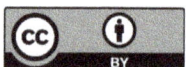

© 2021 by the authors. Licensee MDPI, Basel, Switzerland. This article is an open access article distributed under the terms and conditions of the Creative Commons Attribution (CC BY) license (http://creativecommons.org/licenses/by/4.0/).

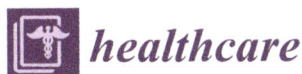

Article

Results of Mentoring in the Psychosocial Well-Being of Young Immigrants and Refugees in Spain

Anna Sánchez-Aragón [1,*], Angel Belzunegui-Eraso [1,2] and Òscar Prieto-Flores [3]

1. Social & Business Research Laboratory (SBRlab), Rovira i Virgili University, 43002 Tarragona, Spain; angel.belzunegui@urv.cat
2. Medical Anthropology Research Center, Rovira i Virgili University, 43002 Tarragona, Spain
3. Department of Pedagogy, School of Education & Psychology, University of Girona, 17071 Girona, Spain; oscar.prieto@udg.edu
* Correspondence: annamaria.sanchez@urv.cat

Received: 12 November 2020; Accepted: 19 December 2020; Published: 24 December 2020

Abstract: This study examined the change processes associated with the Nightingale project, a community-based mentoring programme whose aim is to promote the social inclusion of minors of immigrant origin. A pre-test–post-test study was conducted on a group of 158 young immigrants between the ages of 8 and 15, in which the influence of the mentoring programme on the youths' psychosocial well-being was measured. Non-parametric tests were used to calculate the results before and after mentoring, comparing the results over a six-month period and controlling for sex and age. The analyses reflected associations between mentoring and improvements in specific aspects of the emotional well-being of young immigrants and highlighted the potential of mentorships to cushion the stressful events they are subjected to in the process of adapting to a new social reality.

Keywords: youth mentoring; immigrants; social inclusion; psychosocial well-being; youth health; acculturative stress

1. Introduction

The present study evaluates the effectiveness of the Nightingale mentoring programme in Spain, whose main objective is to promote the social, cultural and linguistic inclusion of students of immigrant origin. The project, which is part of the European-wide Nightingale Mentoring Network, was first carried out in 1997 at the University of Malmö, Sweden; since its success, it has been implemented by twenty-seven other universities in six European countries and one in Africa [1]. The programme is based on the voluntary action of university students who, during the school year, act as mentors of immigrant, refugee or irregular status children and adolescents with the aim of helping them navigate the new educational context and develop a sense of belonging that enables them to find their place within the new country. One key characteristic of the Nightingale project is that both sides benefit: the older person also learns from the younger one and improves their intercultural competence [2].

The Nightingale project is a community-based mentoring programme that fosters relationships of trust between university students and minors of foreign origin with the goal of promoting the positive development of migrants at risk of social exclusion. Throughout the school year, the volunteer mentors work following a one-on-one mentoring scheme to support the youths in their process of integration in the new community. The meetings, which are held weekly, take place outside school hours and last approximately three hours in which the mentor accompanies the minor in acquiring necessary basic elements, such as language and educational guidance. They also aim to expand mentees' social support network outside the school by organising activities with other mentees who are in the same situation and help them to discover the cultural and leisure activities that the new environment offers. For example, some branches of the Nightingale programme teach their mentors in the training sessions how to establish meaningful conversations with their mentees in order to identify adults from their everyday life (i.e., teachers) who can become natural mentors. They are also encouraged to speak in Catalan or Basque if this is not an obstacle for communication or for establishing a close relationship. Through this relationship, the programme helps to support greater social participation of the minors as it helps them to make use of social and community resources, such as public transport and the local library. This is especially beneficial for minors with introverted personalities, so that their mentoring relation provides them with opportunities to reduce their isolation and be more sociable.

Primary and secondary school teachers are in charge of selecting the minors who will receive mentoring. The selection criteria are that (a) they have arrived recently or are of foreign origin but are capable of minimally communicating with others; (b) they lack relationships with adults in their new environment; (c) they are the first generation in their family to have access to university; and (d) they do not start from an extreme level of vulnerability that requires the intervention of a professional rather than a volunteer [1]. With regard to the selection of the mentors, given that the protection of young people is critical, this was carried out through an interview or questionnaire in some cases; and, if selected, an intensive training course of about ten hours was provided [1,3]. The training sessions include the treatment of the cultural diversity and social integration of adolescent immigrants, as well as the collection and exchange of previous mentoring experiences so that the participants are aware of the challenges involved. The primary goal is to build a supportive friendly relationship that facilitates meaningful conversation. For this to happen, the volunteer students are encouraged to mention in their meetings important issues related to the future, the process of integration in the new community or the mentees' relationship with their parents [1]. In return for being mentors, the volunteers receive between one and four ECTS (European Credit Transfer and Accumulation System) credits, depending on the university.

The Nightingale project has been recognised as a successful initiative for vulnerable migrants in Europe [4] and in fact, in Spain, there are already several regions in which it is being carried out, such as Barcelona, Tarragona, Girona, Guipúzcoa and Navarra. The results of this study complement previous evaluations that attribute positive impacts to the programme in terms of academic attitudes—behaviour and dedication to study—and educational expectations, as well as improvements in the minors' communication skills and self-esteem [1,3].

This article gathers together, first of all, the main contributions of the scientific literature regarding the most significant benefits of social support during the migration process. Specifically, it addresses those aspects of mentoring that influence the subjective well-being and health of young people of immigrant origin. Second, it presents the research methodology, followed by a description of the extracted results. The discussion section then offers an interpretation of the findings in light of the available evidence. Finally, the limitations and conclusions of the study are presented.

2. Mentoring with Vulnerable Adolescents

2.1. The Function of Integration in a New Social Reality

There are many scientific studies that highlight the role that non-parental adults can play in the social inclusion of the most vulnerable collectives. The need to improve the support network of people at risk of exclusion has given rise in recent years to formal mentoring programmes, which provide a safe context for the development of relationships. The fundamental goal is to provide support for people who do not usually come into contact with natural mentors or that lack the necessary social skills to identify and form this type of supportive relationship on their own. With this goal in mind, for the formal mentoring the programme recruits adult volunteers to provide friendship, guidance and support to those who most need it. While it is true that the mentoring that arises from natural networks of support usually lasts longer, with stronger affective bonds that last an average of almost a decade [5], formal mentoring has proven to be especially beneficial for those specific groups of minors and adolescents facing risks and adversity. However, not all people have a support network that can help them succeed. Erikson, McDonald and Elder [6] draw attention to the scarcity or absence of social capital in at-risk groups, some from poor communities where low levels of support can be exacerbated by an inability of adults to effectively connect the young people to opportunities that may significantly improve their life journeys.

The results of the scientific evaluations that have been carried out to date highlight that youth mentoring is related to better physical and mental health, as well as to fewer symptoms of depression or suicidal thoughts among young people [5]. An extensive body of research shows that the programmes increase the self-esteem [7,8] and personal satisfaction of the mentee [3] in addition to reducing their levels of stress and anxiety, which is particularly important when it comes to immigrants or refugees, some of them in an irregular situation, who have just arrived to the country and are under great stress due to the integration process in which they find themselves [9,10]. The scientific literature has also reported good results regarding social competencies and communication skills [8]. Studies show that a close bond with the mentor causes participants to develop more positive expectations about relationships with people in their environment, with their parents or friends, and to improve their quality [8,11,12]. This emotional stability is associated with improvements in academic performance and self-efficiency [13], as well as a reduction in behavioural problems such as aggression [14], substance use [15] or delinquent behaviour [16]. As a result, mentoring programmes for minors and young people have grown in popularity as an effective intervention strategy for the social inclusion, health and well-being of the most vulnerable collectives [17]. In the United States, an estimated 2.5 million children and adolescents maintain formal mentoring relationships each year [18].

2.2. Social Support as a Source of Protection Against Stress

The migration process entails an adaption effort whose intensity can be an additional risk factor for developing mental, social or behavioural health problems. The acculturative stress related to cultural differences and perceived racial discrimination in the new country increases the probabilities of young immigrants suffering from anxiety, depression and other mental conditions [19,20], such as eating disorders [21] and alcohol consumption [22]. Refugees, in particular, run a greater risk of suffering symptoms of posttraumatic stress due to exposure to war, long-term persecution or the loss of relatives both in their country of origin and during displacement [23]. Accumulated research has shown that young immigrants and refugees usually have worse mental health than the host population as a result of the challenges of the adaptation process which, as well as forcing them to adhere to new customs and sociocultural codes, is accompanied by changes and distress that occur on an individual level, such as separation from the family as well as from friends and close relationships, the loss of their ethnocultural surroundings, the learning of a new language and the prolongation of uncertainties about their migration status.

These young people suffer from specific vulnerabilities and stress that require people to support them in a lasting way and remain at their side during the adaptation process. Mentoring initiatives are designed to facilitate practical help and advice that enables the minors to cope as best as they can in the new environment; for example, introducing them to local cultural characteristics and recreational opportunities. In Australia, Singh and Tregale [24] observed how mentoring improved participants' access to the networks of social and cultural capital networks. During the programme, the mentors acted as agents for the empowerment of immigrant minors in a process through which the mentees acquired tools to gain autonomy in the new country and achieve life goals. In Europe, Raithelhuber [25] reached similar results and found that mentoring served as a springboard for the efficient integration of the youths participating in the study, unaccompanied refugees who, thanks to their mentors, saw their opportunities for civic participation increase. In the North American context, other studies corroborated both the more practical and instrumental effects of mentoring, such as learning the new language, improving academic performance or the acquisition of social skills [26], and the more emotional effects. For example, Gonzales, Suárez-Orozco and Dedios-Sanguineti [10] recognised that mentoring is especially helpful in reducing the levels of stress and anxiety of illegal immigrant adolescents, which also has a direct impact on reducing school dropout. However, there are still few empirical studies that shed light on the impact of mentoring programmes on the social inclusion of immigrant and refugee adolescents. This study aimed to address this knowledge gap in this particular area.

2.3. Relationship with Parents and Family Dynamics

Empirical evidence shows that minors adapt to the new cultural context faster than their parents. The integration process for adult immigrants or refugees is fraught with difficulties given the deterioration in cognitive flexibility and their solidified ethnicity [27]. This acculturation gap between parents and children increases generational conflicts, sometimes due to the concern of the elderly for the loss of the culture of origin. Perreira, Chapman and Stein [28], through their interviews with Latino migrants with residency in the United States, highlighted parents' concern and unease over the dissolution of cultural heritage and their sons and daughters' adoption of the values, norms and conduct of the majority culture. These differences in the adaptation process leave immigrant minors at a crossroads: on the one hand, they must learn the language and the cultural codes of the new country if they wish to thrive and be successful at school; while on the other hand, they are forced to retain the culture of origin in order to ward off conflict and continue maintaining positive relationships with their co-ethnic families and friends [29,30].

Paradoxically, the rapid acquisition of the vehicular languages causes these young people to take on responsibilities similar to those of the adults in the household, like answering phone calls, helping parents to fill out a job application or acting as interpreters in the doctor's surgery. In primary education, there is a strong assimilative pressure in which the language of instruction is Spanish, and only in the case of the autonomous communities, Catalan and Basque. As a result, the acquisition of vehicular languages is usually even faster in minors. One of the terms that has been used to describe this phenomenon is that of child language brokering [31], which is associated with higher levels of child stress and an increase in family conflicts [32]. In this context, or in others where the young people do not receive sufficient support from their parents due to the family structure or circumstances, mentoring can be a valuable source of support. The research of Dolan et al. [33] on the Big Brothers Big Sisters programme in Ireland supports this theory. After a study of around one hundred and fifty minors, the researchers discovered that mentoring was more beneficial for young people of single-parent families than for those who lived with both parents. After eighteen months, the difference in outcomes between the two groups with regards to perceived support decreased steadily, demonstrating that mentoring can make up for the support that some young people lack.

2.4. Adolescents at Risk, Mentoring and Educational Success

Some research has shown the benefits of mentoring with regards to learning and continuity of studies. For example, in the North American context, Erikson, McDonald and Elder [6] observed how young people from disadvantaged backgrounds who received the support of a non-parental adult were more likely to enrol in a university. The availability of sources of help has been associated with academic success [34,35]. In particular, the presence of a mentor has shown that it can reduce a student's absenteeism, promote a sense of belonging to the school and improve educational expectations [36]. Herrera, Grossman, Kauh and McMaken [13] emphasise that learning difficulties and the intensity with which they experience situations of risk and precariousness can push immigrant minors to processes of demotivation and disaffection with school that lead to educational failure. However, the accumulated evidence indicates that mentoring relationships can reverse this situation and constitute a strong antidote to the dropout rate of immigrant minors and adolescents.

Young people are able to glimpse their future selves in their mentors who, with their experience, provide them with clear and generally positive messages about their own possibilities of success [37]. In the aforementioned research, Singh and Tregale [24] observed how the school motivation of young immigrants and refugee families improved after mentoring, as they saw in their older mentors where higher education could lead them to in the future. In a similar vein, based on their extensive literature review, Larose and Tarabulsy [38] indicated that youth mentoring—even though it takes place outside the educational context—helps to improve students' academic attitudes and their relationship with school, which can have a significant positive impact on student performance. In fact, the results of the first representative survey in the United States with adolescents, collected in The Mentoring Effect [39], show that young people at risk of exclusion who have a mentor are 20% more likely to complete their studies that those who do not. The study of Herrera et al. [13] on the Big Brothers Big Sisters programme shows that mentoring improves the school performance of vulnerable minors, most of them from ethnic minorities, and their perception of their own academic skills.

2.5. Perceived Racial Discrimination and Cultural Mistrust

There are many studies that show the negative psychological and social effects of racial discrimination in the immigrant population [40], especially in those that come from racial and ethnic minorities [41]. The empirical evidence indicates that stress stemming from the feeling of discrimination can—in addition to causing cardiovascular disorders [42]—cause symptoms of anxiety, depression, psychological distress or suicidal ideation that directly affect mental health [43]. Young people who have suffered racialisation first-hand also tend to have greater cultural mistrust of other adults, which can negatively affect different areas of their personal lives. For example, Cooper and Sánchez [44] observed how discrimination, as a subjective perception, with respect to the host society, aggravated the cultural mistrust of Latino boys, which led them to devalue the educational process and lower their academic performance. It has been shown that mentoring can help young people to establish positive intercultural relationships [3,45] and reduce the level of stress stemming from racial discrimination [46]. For this to be possible, the need for culturally aware mentors has been highlighted [47]. It has been demonstrated that adult volunteers who have greater intercultural competencies are more likely to develop greater emotional proximity with the minor and establish a positive relationship that enables the young person to benefit from it [48].

3. Materials and Methods

3.1. Purpose and Design

The purpose of this study was to evaluate the changes in specific aspects of emotional well-being derived from the Nightingale mentoring programme aimed at adolescents of foreign origin in the primary and secondary schools of Barcelona, Tarragona, Girona, Guipúzcoa and Navarra. In order to contribute to the literature on social mentoring, this study examined the effects of mentoring on the psychological well-being of minors of immigrant origin.

The evaluation of some aspects of participants' emotional well-being resulting from applying the programme was performed through a pre-test–post-test design of a single non-randomised group [49,50], with a six-month difference between the first and second data collections on the study's different areas of focus. A longitudinal strategy was chosen through a dynamic comparison, including the repetition of response measures.

Specifically, this assesses aspects related to the mental health of the mentee, their self-esteem and personal satisfaction, as well as their perceptions of social support and racial discrimination during their integration process in the host country.

3.2. Sample

It was not possible to randomise the selection of participants due to the small starting population size, and also because participation required voluntary consent.

The study had a sample of 158 students, between 8 and 15 years of age, 79 (50%) of whom were girls, and with an average age of 12.17 years (Std. Deviation = 1.79). The participants came from different countries, although the majority were from Morocco, Honduras, Gambia, India and the Dominican Republic. Sixty-two percent were first generation immigrants and 38% second generation. Among them, 17.7% arrived in Spain the same year that they began their participation in the programme (2018), 19.6% arrived in 2017, 11.4% between 2014 and 2016, and 13.3% over five years ago (between 2007 and 2013). Moreover, 48.7% of the participants were under 12 years of age; and 51.3% were between 12 and 15. At the time of this study, 51.3% of the minors lived in a nuclear household with their parents; 12% in a household with more than two nuclear families (with extended family); 19.6% in a single-parent family; 3.8% with grandparents or other relatives; and 12.7% in a single-parent household but with other relatives. Participants' characteristics are depicted in Table 1.

Table 1. Composition of the study group.

Study Group	N	Percent
Male	79	50.0
Female	79	50.0
Below 12	77	48.7
12 and above	81	51.3

Source: the authors.

The programme began at the start of the 2018–2019 school year, and the outcomes of the participants were observed during that year. Before the evaluation, the informed consents were given for each father/mother and/or legal guardian, and only after obtaining the corresponding permission were the tests administered.

3.3. Study Variables

The Youth Environment Stressors Index [51] collects the joint scores of the following items, which all refer to events that happened in the previous year: someone close dying; moved or changed home; changed school; a close friend moved away; picked on or bullied at school or in the neighbourhood; parents separated or divorced; parent/guardian stopped working or lost a job; and brother/sister dropped out of school. All the items were categorised as: 1 = Strongly disagree; 2 = Disagree; 3 = Agree; 4 = Strongly agree.

The following questions were used as indicators of stressors: (a) Suddenly scared for no reason?—with answers: 0 = No, 1 = Yes, sometimes; 2 = Often; (b) Feeling blocked in getting things done?—with answers: 0 = No, 1 = Yes, sometimes; 2 = Often.

It is not properly a scale but rather a variable resulting from the summation of a number of items that give each individual a total count of environmental stressors. The resulting variable (total number of environmental stressors endorsed) is used as an ordinal variable and does not need to present the required properties on a scale that tries to measure a coherent dimension [51].

The Cultural Mistrust Index [52] was generated from the summation of the scores to different items: You should be suspicious of the native population from the beginning; You can trust the native population like members of your own group; The native population tend to keep their promises less; The native population tend to be honest with us; The native population tend to say one thing and do another; You should be cautious about what you say because it will be used against you; The native population usually tend to keep their word; The native population tend to feel superior to us. All the items were categorised as: 1 = Strongly disagree; 2 = Disagree; 3 = Agree; 4 = Strongly agree.

This index was developed from a proposal contained in Benkert, Peters, Clark and Keves-Foster [52], who used a more extensive instrument with high internal consistency (Cronbach's alpha = 0.89). In our sample, Cronbach's alpha was 0.89.

The Social Support Index [53] is the result of the summation of the scores of the following items: I have the social support of teachers; I have the social support of friends; I have the social support of parents/guardians; I have social support outside the family and school. All the items were categorised in the same way: 1 = Strongly disagree; 2 = Disagree; 3 = Moderately disagree; 4 = Neutral; 5 = Moderately agree; 6 = Agree; 7 = Strongly agree.

This index was developed from various scales used by Wang and Eccles [53], such as the Teacher Social Support (with a Cronbach's alpha of 0.80), the Peer Social Support (with a Cronbach's alpha of 0.82) and the Parent Social Support (with a Cronbach's alpha of 0.77) scales. In our study, Cronbach's alpha obtained a value of 0.53.

The Self-Esteem Index [54] consists of 10 items that allude to global feelings of self-esteem and self-perception. Five of the items are positive statements: I feel that I'm a person of worth, at least on an equal level with others; I feel that I have a number of good qualities; I am able to do things as well as most other people; I take a positive attitude toward myself; On the whole, I am satisfied with myself—and five others that are negative statements: All in all, I am inclined to feel that I am a failure; I feel I do not have much to be proud of; I wish I could have more respect for myself; I certainly feel useless at times; at times I think I am no good at all. All the items were categorised as: 1 = Strongly disagree; 2 = Disagree; 3 = Agree; 4 = Strongly agree.

The psychometric tests of the scale presented by Rosenberg [54] reflected a reproducibility coefficient of 0.92, which indicates excellent internal consistency. Test–retest reliability over a two-week period revealed correlations of 0.85 and 0.88, which indicates stability. In our analysis, Cronbach's alpha was 0.73.

The Academic Self-Efficacy Index [55] consists of the following items: I feel like I do well in school; It is easy for me to learn most things; Even when I study hard, I cannot do well on tests; When I try hard, I can learn most things; I can get good grades even when I do not try hard; There is no way a student like me can get good grades; and I think I am a smart person. All the items were categorised as: 1 = Very false; 2 = More false than true; 3 = More true than false; 4 = Very true.

In the consistency analysis performed by Owen and Froman [55], for reliability estimation, alpha internal consistency estimates were 0.90. In the analysis of our data, Cronbach's alpha was 0.54.

The Cognitive Engagement Index [56] consists of the following items: With regards to learning at school, how often do the following occur: I enjoy learning new things; I get bored easily with school work; I feel good when I learn something new even when it is hard and I do homework whenever it is required. All the items were categorised as: 1 = Never; 2 = Few times; 3 = Most of the times; 4 = Always. This index was a composite of the variables validated by previous studies, such as Finn and Voelkl [56], observing compliance or the non-compliance of the aforementioned school requirements. This index had a Cronbach's alpha of 0.43.

3.4. Analysis Performed

The lack of randomisation has led to non-parametric analyses to measure the effects. *Wilcoxon (Z) t-tests*—a non-parametric test equivalent to the Student's *t*-test—were carried out to determine whether the programme had an effect on the adolescents. This test was used because the distributions failed to meet the criteria of normality and homoscedasticity, in addition to being based on small subsamples. Most of the measurements that were taken correspond to ordinal variables with few ranges. For each of the Z tests, Cohen's *d* was calculated as the effect size coefficient [57] (p. 12) [58].

4. Results

The results show that the mentored students that took part in the project reduced the impact of stressful life experiences measured through the Youth Environment Stressors Index (Table 2). During the course of the programme (pre-post), they significantly reduced their levels of environmental stress ($Z = 5.931$; $p = 0.000$; $d_{Cohen} = 1.07$). This difference is even greater in the girls ($Z = 4.679$; $p = 0.000$; $d_{Cohen} = 1.238$) than in the boys ($Z = 3.666$; $p = 0.000$; $d_{Cohen} = 0.906$). The differences are also significant if controlled by age.

In addition to environmental stressors, another source of anxiety in children is the interaction with the native population, since it can expose them to more or less subtle prejudices and discrimination. In this regard, the mentoring relationship did not cause the study participants to reduce their attitude of suspicion and feeling of distrust toward others ($Z = -1.090$; $p = 0.276$). No significant differences were observed by either sex or age.

The perceived availability of social support strengthened, in all cases, the psychological well-being of the mentees. The perception of social support increased and this is reflected in a higher score of the Social Support Index for the whole sample ($Z = -6.922$; $p < 0.01$; $d_{Cohen} = 1.319$; Table 2). More specifically, having informal sources of social support correlated negatively with psychological symptoms of stress (Spearman's rho = -0.337; $p = 0.000$; $d_{Cohen} = 0.716$) and positively with the Resilience Index (Spearman's rho = 0.246; $p = 0.002$; $d_{Cohen} = 0.508$), although resilience scores were only significant for the girls ($Z = -1.661$; $p = 0.097$, and as seen when considering a 0.10 error).

Table 2. Non-parametric tests for pre-post measurements.

Measure	N	Mean (Pre)	Mean (Post)	T of Wilcoxon (Z)	p	d_{Cohen}
Social Support Index	158	13.66	18.58	−6.922	0.000	1.319
Boys	79	13.37	17.96	−4.534	0.000	1.186
Girls	79	13.96	19.21	−5.243	0.000	1.461
Below 12	77	14.40	19.50	−4.832	0.000	1.319
12 and above	81	12.96	17.72	−4.907	0.000	1.301
Youth Environment Stressors Index	158	2.37	1.53	5.931	0.000	1.07
Boys	79	2.14	1.51	3.666	0.000	0.906
Girls	79	2.61	1.55	4.679	0.000	1.238
Below 12	77	2.14	1.34	4.334	0.000	1.136
12 and above	81	2.59	1.71	4.150	0.000	1.039
Self-Esteem Index	158	30.67	30.37	0.766	0.444	
I have at least one friend at school to help me with homework	158	3.27	3.63	−2.038	0.042	0.329
Boys	79	3.28	3.41	−0.549	0.583	
Girls	79	3.25	3.85	−2.251	0.024	0.524
Below 12	77	3.26	3.81	−2.171	0.030	0.511
12 and above	81	3.27	3.46	−0.713	0.476	
Someone at school makes me feel successful	158	4.01	4.12	−0.706	0.480	
Boys	79	3.89	3.76	0.917	0.359	
Girls	79	4.13	4.48	−2.003	0.045	0.463
Below 12	77	4.09	4.44	−1.807	0.071	0.421
12 and above	81	3.93	3.81	0.698	0.485	
I would prefer to go to another school						
12 and above	81	4.64	4.35	2.834	0.005	0.664
Academic Self-Efficacy Index	158	20.28	22.62	−7.693	0.000	1.548
Boys	79	19.97	22.51	−5.905	0.000	1.778
Girls	79	20.59	22.73	−5.088	0.000	1.396
Below 12	77	20.30	23.27	−6.631	0.000	2.308
12 and above	81	20.27	22.00	−4.178	0.000	1.048
Cognitive Engagement Index	158	9.22	9.48	−1.956	0.051	
Boys	79	9.18	9.33	−0.963	0.336	
Girls	79	9.27	9.63	−1.733	0.083	
Below 12	77	9.21	9.57	−2.088	0.037	0.054
12 and above	81	9.23	9.40	−0.755	0.450	

Source: the authors.

After six months, the group of adolescents perceived greater social support from their local network, especially the girls and those under 12 that had more diverse sources of help after the intervention (Table 2). Both of these groups found social support networks in the school and stated having at least one classmate that helped them with the homework (girls group: $Z = -2.251$; $p = 0.024$; $d_{Cohen} = 0.524$; under 12 group: $Z = -2.171$; $p = 0.030$; $d_{Cohen} = 0.511$; Table 2). This tangible support, which includes physical acts of help and educational support in schoolwork, was not the only kind of support they received. The support of self-esteem, related to recognising their personal worth, was also perceived by these mentees in the school, where they assured: "Someone at school makes me feel successful" (girls group: $Z = -2.003$; $p = 0.045$; $d_{Cohen} = 0.463$; under 12 group: $Z = -1.807$; $p = 0.071$; $d_{Cohen} = 0.421$; Table 2).

Regarding school dynamics, the results showed that the Nightingale project was associated with more positive attitudes of the mentees towards the school and their peers, specifically for the over-twelves group, who significantly improved their response to the item: "I would prefer to go another school" ($Z = 2.834$; $p = 0.005$; $d_{Cohen} = 0.664$; Table 2).

This connection has helped those adolescents who participated in mentoring to improve academically (Table 2). The pre-test–post-test shows an improvement in the Academic Self-Efficacy Index for the participants as a whole ($Z = -7.693$; $p = 0.000$; $d_{Cohen} = 1.548$). This improvement is greater in the group of boys ($Z = -5.905$; $p = 0.000$; $d_{Cohen} = 1.778$) and in the children under 12 ($Z = -6.631$; $p = 0.000$; $d_{Cohen} = 2.308$).

With regard to self-esteem, no changes were observed between pre-test and post-test for the whole sample ($Z = 0.766$; $p = 0.444$; Table 2), nor for boys and girls separately. Statistical significance was only observed in those over twelve years of age, whose self-esteem increased ($Z = 1.968$; $p = 0.049$; $d_{Cohen} = 0.448$). However, when controlled for age (under 12 years and over 12 years), mentoring was positively associated with the adolescents' assessment of their abilities and degree of personal satisfaction. This improvement in self-concept occurred in the oldest participants in the positive responses to the items used in the questionnaires: "I feel that I am a person of worth, at least on an equal level with others" ($Z = -2.466$; $p = 0.014$; $d_{Cohen} = 0.569$) and "I am able to do things as well as most other people" ($Z = -2.376$; $p = 0.018$; $d_{Cohen} = 0.547$). This correlates with an improvement in the Cognitive Engagement Index score for the children under 12, the only group in which there are statistically significant differences between the pre-test and post-test scores ($Z = -2.088$; $p = 0.037$; $d_{Cohen} = 0.054$; Table 2).

5. Discussion

This research aimed to identify whether the presence of a mentor that provides support can improve some specific aspects of the social and emotional well-being of young immigrants. The results of this study show that the development of a mentoring relationship improved some aspects of the psychosocial well-being of young immigrants and refugees, protecting them from the negative impact of the stress involved in adapting to a new country. This finding is consistent with earlier research that shows that the presence of a non-parental adult acts as a support that helps mentees increase their ability to overcome adverse events, such as those arising from leaving and adapting to a new context [26].

The support of a reliable ally provided participants with a number of personal and social benefits insofar as it helped them weave local support networks. Some of these benefits involve an improvement in their emotional and cognitive skills, as well as better social development. The mentees that participated in the project, as has been observed in other participants of formal mentoring programmes aimed at the inclusion of young people of foreign origin [25,59], improved their access to social capital resources, whose social networks constitute the framework in which support exchanges take place. The perceived availability of social support reduced some symptoms of stress associated with the migration process and made the youths more resilient, despite enduring significant adversity. The impact of mentoring on the promotion of resilience in adolescents from ethnic minorities supports the findings of a recent literature review [36,60–62].

Participation in the Nightingale project improved the minors' relationships with their classmates. This corroborates the results of previous research that shows a positive association between mentoring and peer relationship development [63]. The importance of close peer relationships for immigrant adolescents has been found in previous social science research [64,65], the results of which show that peer social support not only promotes adaptation to the host country but also contributes to greater psychological well-being. In the present study, the increase in the perception of social support in school, as well as providing mentees with educational support, strengthened their feeling of personal worth.

The Nightingale project generated significant positive changes in the minors, which helped them in their process of adaptation to the school. During the intervention, the participants improved social relationships with their classmates and also showed more assertive attitudes towards the school and teachers. These results coincide with those found by various authors [13,66], which show the effectiveness of mentoring programmes to promote a positive change in a student's attitude towards the school. This inner transformation is vital to help adolescent immigrants and refugees to improve their academic performance. Over the course of the programme, the students' psychological involvement in learning—cognitive commitment—increased significantly. This difference in the pre-test–post-test intervention, as other authors have suggested [3,24], might be due to the positive role model provided by the mentors. The Nightingale project volunteers are young undergraduates who, because of their status as students, can foster the minors' motivation during their transition to post-compulsory education.

In contrast to other research on informal or 'natural' mentoring relationships [46,67], no evidence was found showing the programme's impact on the reduction in perceived racial discrimination. It is possible that in order for mentors to moderate the attitude of suspicion and feeling of mistrust towards others, the mentor needs to focus on responding to this specific goal—for example, through specific conversations on discriminatory experiences. This was not assessed in the study.

6. Limitations

One limitation of this study was that the sample was not randomly selected, which precludes making generalisable statements about mentoring processes that include the immigrant population. This study was based on a single group, pre-test–post-test design, without a control group. The objective was to measure certain changes in the emotional well-being of young people, and it is therefore not an impact analysis of the project as it does not have a comparative reference in a group on which the activity has not been developed. One limitation that should be taken into account is the effect that other non-controlled variables may have had on the observed changes in some aspects of the emotional well-being of young people. The non-experimental pre-test–post-test design does not manage to control confounding variables that might exert some influence on the results. This limitation will be addressed in a second phase of the study, which will incorporate a qualitative analysis of interviews with mentees in which information will be collected about their perception of mentoring in their emotional states. The main difficulty will be that of differentiating the specific effects of the programme from those non-specific effects that derive from the lack of comparability of the group with a control group, which compromises the internal validity of the study. Therefore, causal effects are not deduced from this analysis; rather, the differences in variability in scores need to be understood as possible effects derived from the intervention. In fact, this type of design is not exempt from the Hawthorne effect; that is, the responses may have been induced by the participants' knowledge that they are being studied.

Nor do the participants represent all the geographical areas where the Nightingale programme is implemented, which means that these results cannot be extrapolated to the mentees that take part in other universities around Europe (Sweden, Norway, Austria, Switzerland, etc.) and Africa (Ghana).

Furthermore, the use of self-report questionnaires structured on Likert-type scales made it difficult to carry out a more precise evaluation, as the participants gave their own meanings and interpretations. While this method allowed a very wide range of effects to be explored—many of which were inaccessible to direct observation—in a relatively short time, the use of this methodology prevented the appearance of emerging categories on the nature of the relationships and their effects. To increase the validity of the measures, we recommend that future evaluations be conducted with multiple sources, for example gathering the testimonies of parents and teachers, and through the use of the multimethod perspective or multiple approaches that facilitate the possibility of studying mentoring relationships quantitatively and qualitatively.

One additional limitation, which could explain the moderate effect of the programme, is the length of the study. Some research points out that the minimum time it takes to build a trusting relationship is six months [68]. It has also been shown that the longer and more trusting the mentoring relationship, the greater the impact capacity of the programmes [69].

Finally, it should be noted that for certain instruments used, the measurement value of their consistency was below the standard values, a fact that that must be taken into account when drawing conclusions, and that necessitates the continued improvement of the instruments applied to the case of mentoring.

7. Conclusions

The results of this study provide empirical evidence of the positive effects of social support on the emotional well-being of young immigrants and refugees. Specifically, the potential of mentoring programmes to cushion the stressful events to which they are subjected is made evident. The social support perceived during the Nightingale project contributed to improve some aspects related to the psychological well-being of the mentees, who saw their levels of personal satisfaction increase in a short period of time.

The data gleaned from this study suggest that mentoring is associated with more positive indices of personal well-being, although it can produce different effects in women and men, as a review of the relevant literature has shown [63,70]. While scientific research has increasingly focused on observing the effects of mentoring on social inclusion, empirical work addressing the influence of sex on the process and impact of such a relationship is scarce and mostly comes from studies on school-based mentoring programmes [66,71,72]. Therefore, interdisciplinary work with a gender perspective is needed that can address the gaps that remain in the evaluation of youth mentoring and its effects differentiated by sex.

The results reveal the importance of school counsellors, psychologists and social workers providing immigrant minors with programmes that encourage the building of social networks and the promotion of social support. We believe that prioritising policies and services that ensure a socially supportive environment in the reception of young people of foreign origin may help reduce the stressors associated with the migration process, which place minors in a vulnerable situation. The post-mentoring outcomes support the scientific consensus in the field of youth mentoring regarding the key role that relationships with non-parental adults play in supporting the social inclusion and subjective well-being of young immigrants.

With the aim of promoting the implementation of social mentoring programmes in schools, the findings of this study will be presented to primary and secondary school teachers. Educational institutions must show concern about the reality of students of foreign origin, at risk of exclusion, so as to help them overcome the adversities that arise from the adaptation process, avoiding leaving scars that affect emotional stability and lead to poor academic performance. From what is stated in this study, it can be seen that there is a need to promote the implementation of mentoring programmes as a reception plan that fosters the development of supportive relationships between adults and minors that serve the latter as a resource to try to adapt to the new environment, learn the language, build local networks and plan for the future.

Author Contributions: Conceptualisation, A.S.-A., A.B.-E. and Ò.P.-F.; methodology, A.S.-A., A.B.-E. and Ò.P.-F.; validation, A.S.-A., A.B.-E. and Ò.P.-F.; formal analysis, A.S.-A. and A.B.-E.; resources and data curation, Ò.P.-F.; writing—original draft preparation, A.S.-A.; writing—review and editing, A.S.-A., A.B.-E. and Ò.P.-F.; funding acquisition, A.B.-E. and Ò.P.-F. All authors have read and agreed to the published version of the manuscript.

Funding: This research was funded by the Secretariat of Universities and Research of the Government of Catalonia's Ministry of Business and Knowledge, the European Union and European Social Fund. (FSE) (2020 FI-B1 00109).

Institutional Review Board Statement: The study was conducted according to the guidelines of the Declaration of Helsinki, and approved by the Institutional Review Board (or Ethics Committee) of the University of Girona under the code: CEBRU0001-2018 (6th of April 2018).

Informed Consent Statement: Informed consent was obtained from the parents of all subjects involved in the study as well as their assent.

Data Availability Statement: The data presented in this study are openly available in Harvard Dataserve repository at https://doi.org/10.7910/DVN/ZXC8RC.

Acknowledgments: This study is part of the Project RECERCAIXA2017UdG, Applying Mentoring: Social and technological innovations for the social inclusion of immigrants and refugees, funded by the RecerCaixa programme, a collaboration of "La Caixa" Welfare Projects and the Catalan Association of Public Universities. We would also like to express our gratitude to the Chair for Social Inclusion of Rovira i Virgili University for its assistance.

Conflicts of Interest: The authors declare no conflict of interest.

References

1. Prieto-Flores, O.; Casademont, X.; Feu, J. "I had him in my head reminding me to persist": The Role of Mentoring in Shaping Immigrant Youth Expectations. *Pedagog. Treb. Soc. Rev. Ciències Soc. Apl.* **2019**, *8*, 3–25. [CrossRef]
2. Sild-Lönroth, C. *The Nightingale Scheme—A Song for the Heart*; Malmö University: Malmö, Sweden, 2007.
3. Feu, J. How an intervention Project contributes to social inclusion of adolescents and young people of foreign origin. *Child. Youth Serv. Rev.* **2015**, *52*, 144–149. [CrossRef]
4. Delvino, M.; Spencer, S. *Migrants with Irregular Status in Europe: Guidance for Municipalities*; University of Oxford: Oxford, UK, 2019.
5. DuBois, D.L.; Silverthorn, N. Characteristics of natural mentoring relationships and adolescent adjustment: Evidence from a national study. *Am. J. Public Health* **2005**, *95*, 518–524. [CrossRef] [PubMed]
6. Erikson, L.D.; McDonald, S.; Elder, G.H., Jr. Informal mentors and education: Complementary or compensatory resources? *Sociol. Educ.* **2009**, *82*, 344–367. [CrossRef] [PubMed]
7. Marino, C.; Santinello, M.; Lenzi, M.; Santoro, P.; Bergamin, M.; Gaboardi, M.; Calcagnì, A.; Altoè, G.; Perkins, D.D. Can mentoring promote self-esteem and school connectedness? An evaluation of the mentor-UP project. *Psychosoc. Interv.* **2019**, *29*, 1–8. [CrossRef]
8. Karcher, M.J. The effects of developmental mentoring and high school mentors' attendance on their younger mentees' self-esteem, social skills, and connectedness. *Psychol. Sch.* **2005**, *42*, 65–77. [CrossRef]
9. Oberoi, A.K. *Mentoring for First-Generation Immigrant and Refugee Youth*; National Mentoring Resource Center: Boston, MA, USA, 2006.
10. Gonzales, R.G.; Suárez-Orozco, C.; Dedios-Sanguineti, M.C. No place to belong: Contextualizing concepts of mental health among undocumented immigrant youth in the United States. *Am. Behav. Sci.* **2013**, *57*, 1174–1199. [CrossRef]
11. DuBois, D.L.; Neville, H.A.; Parra, G.R.; Pugh-Lilly, A.O. Testing a new model of mentoring. In *A Critical View of Youth Mentoring. New Directions for Youth Development: Theory, Research, and Practice*; Noam, G.G., Rhodes, J.E., Eds.; Jossey-Bass: San Francisco, CA, USA, 2002; Volume 93, pp. 21–57.
12. Spencer, R.; Drew, A.L.; Horn, J.P.; Gowdy, G.; Rhodes, J.E. "A positive guiding hand:" A qualitative examination of Youth-Initiated Mentoring and the promotion of interdependence among foster care youth. *Child. Youth Serv. Rev.* **2018**, *93*, 41–50. [CrossRef]
13. Herrera, C.; Grossman, J.B.; Kauh, T.J.; McMaken, J. Mentoring in schools: An impact study of Big Brothers Big Sisters school-based mentoring. *Child Dev.* **2011**, *82*, 346–361. [CrossRef]
14. Jolliffe, D.; Farrington, D.P. A Rapid Evidence Assessment of the Impact of Mentoring Re-Offending: A Summary. Cambridge University: Home Office Online Report 11/07. Available online: https://www.youthmentoring.org.nz/content/docs/Home_Office_Impact_of_mentoring.pdf (accessed on 26 October 2020).
15. Rhodes, J.E.; Reddy, R.; Grossman, J.B. The protective influence of mentoring on adolescents' substance use: Direct and indirect pathways. *Appl. Dev. Sci.* **2005**, *9*, 31–47. [CrossRef]

16. Heller, S.B.; Shah, A.K.; Guryan, J.; Ludwig, J.; Mullainathan, S.; Pollack, H.A. Thinking, fast and slow? Some field experiments to reduce crime and dropout in Chicago. *Q. J. Econ.* **2017**, *132*, 1–54. [CrossRef] [PubMed]
17. Preston, J.M.; Prieto-Flores, O.; Rhodes, J.E. Mentoring in context: A comparative study of youth mentoring programs in the United States and continental Europe. *Youth Soc.* **2019**, *51*, 900–914. [CrossRef]
18. Raposa, E.B.; Dietz, N.; Rhodes, J.E. Trends in volunteer mentoring in the United States: Analysis of a decade of census survey data. *Am. J. Community Psychol.* **2017**, *59*, 3–14. [CrossRef] [PubMed]
19. Sirin, S.R.; Ryce, P.; Gupta, T.; Rogers-Sirin, L. The role of acculturative stress on mental health symptoms for immigrant adolescents: A longitudinal investigation. *Dev. Psychol.* **2013**, *49*, 736–748. [CrossRef]
20. Sirin, S.R.; Rogers-Sirin, L.; Cressen, J.; Gupta, T.; Ahmed, S.F.; Novoa, A.D. Discrimination-related stress effects on the development of internalizing symptoms among Latino adolescents. *Child Dev.* **2015**, *86*, 709–725. [CrossRef]
21. Simmons, S.; Limbers, C.A. Acculturative stress and emotional eating in Latino adolescents. *Eat Weight Disord.* **2019**, *24*, 905–914. [CrossRef]
22. Oshri, A.; Schwartz, S.; Unger, J.; Kwon, J.; Des Rosiers, S.; Baezconde-Garbanati, L.E. Bicultural stress, identity formation, and alcohol expectancies and misuse in Hispanic adolescents: A developmental approach. *J. Youth Adolesc.* **2014**, *43*, 2054–2068. [CrossRef]
23. Comisión Española de Ayuda al Refugiado (CEAR). *Informe 2018: Las Personas Refugiadas en España y Europa*; Comisión Española de Ayuda al Refugiado (CEAR): Madrid, Spain, 2018; Available online: https://www.cear.es/wp-content/uploads/2018/06/Informe-CEAR-2018.pdf (accessed on 28 August 2020).
24. Singh, S.; Tregale, R. From homeland to home: Widening participation through the LEAP-Macquarie Mentoring (Refugee Mentoring) Program. *Int. Stud. Widening Particip.* **2015**, *2*, 15–27.
25. Raithelhuber, E. 'If we want, they help us in any way': How 'unaccompanied refugee minors' experience mentoring relationships. *Eur. J. Soc. Work* **2019**. [CrossRef]
26. Rotich, J. Mentoring as a springboard to acculturation of immigrant students into American schools. *J. Case Stud. Educ.* **2011**, *1*, 1–8.
27. Birman, D.; Morland, L. Immigrant and refugee youth. In *Handbook of Youth Mentoring*, 2nd ed.; DuBois, D.L., Karcher, M.J., Eds.; Sage: Thousand Oaks, CA, USA, 2014; pp. 355–368.
28. Perreira, K.M.; Chapman, M.V.; Stein, G.L. Becoming an American parent: Overcoming challenges and finding strengths in a new immigrant Latino community. *J. Fam. Issues* **2006**, *27*, 1383–1414. [CrossRef]
29. Birman, D. Acculturation gap and family adjustment: Findings with Soviet Jewish refugees in the United States and implications for measurement. *J. Cross-Cult. Psychol.* **2006**, *37*, 568–589. [CrossRef]
30. Birman, D.; Trickett, E.; Buchanan, R.M. A tale of two cities: Replication of a study on the acculturation and adaptation of immigrant adolescents from the Former Soviet Union in a different community context. *Am. J. Community Psychol.* **2005**, *35*, 83–101. [CrossRef] [PubMed]
31. Antonini, R. Child language brokering. In *Routledge Encyclopedia of Interpreting Studies*; Pochhacker, F., Ed.; Routledge: London, UK, 2015; p. 48.
32. Jones, C.; Trickett, E.; Birman, D. Determinants and consequences of child culture brokering in families from the former Soviet Union. *Am. J. Community Psychol.* **2012**, *50*, 182–196. [CrossRef] [PubMed]
33. Dolan, P.; Brady, B.; O Regan, C.; Canavan, J.; Russell, D.; Forkan, C. *Big Brothers Big Sisters (BBBS) of Ireland: Evaluation Study. Report 3: Summary Report*; UNESCO Child and Family Research Centre on behalf of Foróige: Galway, Ireland, 2011. [CrossRef]
34. Suárez-Orozco, C.; Pimentel, A.; Martin, M. The significance of relationships: Academic engagement and achievement among newcomer immigrant youth. *Teach. Coll. Rec.* **2009**, *111*, 712–749.
35. Green, G.; Rhodes, J.; Hirsch, A.H.; Suárez-Orozco, C.; Camic, P.M. Supportive adult relationships and the academic attainment of Latin American immigrant youth. *J. Sch. Psychol.* **2008**, *46*, 393–412. [CrossRef]
36. Sánchez, B.; Esparza, P.; Colón, Y. Natural mentoring under the microscope: An investigation of mentoring relationships and Latino adolescents' academic adjustment. *J. Community Psychol.* **2008**, *36*, 468–482. [CrossRef]
37. Zirkel, S. Is there a place for me? Role models and academic identity among White students and students of color. *Teach. Coll. Rec.* **2002**, *104*, 357–376. [CrossRef]

38. Larose, S.; Tarabulsy, G. Acadamically at-risk students. In *Handbook of Youth Mentoring*; DuBois, D.L., Karcher, M.J., Eds.; Sage: Thousand Oaks, CA, USA, 2005; pp. 440–453.
39. Bruce, M.; Bridgeland, J. The Mentoring Effect: Young People's Perspectives on the Outcomes and Availability of Mentoring. Washington, D.C.: Civic Enterprises with Hart Research Associates for MENTOR: The National Mentoring Partnership. 2014. Available online: https://files.eric.ed.gov/fulltext/ED558065.pdf (accessed on 6 July 2020).
40. Szaflarski, M.; Bauldry, S. The Effects of Perceived Discrimination on Immigrant and Refugee Physical and Mental Health. *Adv. Med. Sociol.* **2019**, *19*, 173–204. [CrossRef]
41. Colen, C.G.; Ramey, D.M.; Cooksey, E.C.; Williams, D.R. Racial disparities in health among nonpoor African Americans and Hispanics: The role of acute and chronic discrimination. *Soc. Sci. Med.* **2017**, *199*, 167–180. [CrossRef]
42. Panza, G.A.; Puhl, R.M.; Taylor, B.A.; Zaleski, A.L.; Livingston, J.; Pescatello, L.S. Links between discrimination and cardiovascular health among socially stigmatized groups: A systematic review. *PLoS ONE* **2019**, *14*, e0217623. [CrossRef] [PubMed]
43. Hwang, W.-C.; Goto, S. The impact of perceived racial discrimination on the mental health of Asian American and Latino college students. *Cult. Divers. Ethn. Minority Psychol.* **2008**, *14*, 326–335. [CrossRef] [PubMed]
44. Cooper, A.C.; Sánchez, B. The roles of racial discrimination, cultural mistrust and gender in Latina/o school attitudes and academic achievement. *J. Res. Adolesc.* **2016**, *26*, 1036–1047. [CrossRef] [PubMed]
45. Pryce, J.M.; Silverthorn, N.; Sanchez, B.; DuBois, D.L. GirlPOWER! Strengthening mentoring relationships through a structured, gender-specific program. *New Dir. Youth Dev.* **2010**, *126*, 89–105. [CrossRef] [PubMed]
46. Griffith, A.N.; Hurd, N.M.; Hussain, S.B. "I didn't come to school for this": A qualitative examination of experiences with race-related stressors and coping responses among Black students attending a predominantly White Institution. *J. Adolesc. Res.* **2019**, *34*, 115–139. [CrossRef]
47. Griffiths, M.; Sawrikar, P.; Muir, K. Culturally appropriate mentoring for Horn of African young people in Australia. *Youth Stud. Aust.* **2009**, *28*, 32–40.
48. Sánchez, B.; Colón-Torres, Y.; Feuer, R.; Roundfield, K.E.; Berardi, L. Race, ethnicity and culture in mentoring relationships. In *Handbook of Youth Mentoring*, 2nd ed.; DuBois, D.L., Karcher, M.J., Eds.; Sage: Thousand Oaks, CA, USA, 2014; pp. 145–158.
49. Campbell, D.; Stanley, J. *Diseños Experimentales y Cuasi-Experimentales en la Investigación Social*; Amorrortu: Buenos Aires, Argentina, 2011.
50. Dimitrov, D.M.; Rumrill, J.; Phillip, D. Pretest-posttest designs and measurement of change. *Work* **2003**, *20*, 159–165.
51. Raposa, E.B.; Rhodes, J.E.; Herrera, C. The impact of youth risk on mentoring relationship quality: Do mentor characteristics matter? *Am. J. Community Psychol.* **2016**, *57*, 320–329. [CrossRef]
52. Benkert, R.; Peters, R.M.; Clark, R.; Keves-Foster, K. Effects of perceived racism, cultural mistrust and trust in providers on satisfaction with care. *J. Natl. Med. Assoc.* **2006**, *98*, 1532–1540.
53. Wang, M.-T.; Eccles, J.S. Social Support Matters: Longitudinal Effects of Social Support on Three Dimensions of School Engagement from Middle to High School. *Child Dev.* **2012**, *83*, 877–895. [CrossRef]
54. Rosenberg, M. *Society and the Adolescent Self-Image*; Princeton University Press: Princeton, NJ, USA, 1965.
55. Owen, S.V.; Froman, R.D. Development of a College Academic Self-Efficacy Scale. Reports Research/Technical (143). In Proceedings of the Annual Meeting of the National Council on Measurement in Education, New Orleans, LA, USA, 6–8 April 1988; Available online: https://files.eric.ed.gov/fulltext/ED298158.pdf (accessed on 28 November 2020).
56. Finn, J.D.; Voelkl, K.E. School characteristics related to student engagement. *J. Negro Educ.* **1993**, *62*, 249–268. [CrossRef]
57. Fritz, C.O.; Morris, P.E.; Richler, J.J. Effect size estimates: Current use, calculations, and interpretation. *J. Exp. Psychol. Gen.* **2012**, *141*, 2–18. [CrossRef] [PubMed]
58. Cohen, B. *Explaining Psychological Statistics*, 3rd ed.; John Wiley: New York, NY, USA, 2008.

59. Shier, M.L.; Gouthro, S.; de Goias, R.D. The pursuit of social capital among adolescent high school aged girls: The role of formal mentor-mentee relationships. *Child. Youth Serv. Rev.* **2018**, *93*, 276–282. [CrossRef]
60. Wittrup, A.R.; Hussain, S.B.; Albright, J.N.; Hurd, N.M.; Varner, F.A.; Mattis, J.S. Natural mentors, racial pride, and academic engagement among black adolescents: Resilience in the context of perceived discrimination. *Youth Soc.* **2016**, *51*, 463–483. [CrossRef]
61. Hurd, N.M.; Zimmerman, M.A. Natural mentoring relationships among adolescent mothers: A study of resilience. *J. Res. Adolesc.* **2010**, *20*, 789–809. [CrossRef]
62. Hurd, N.M.; Zimmerman, M.A. Natural mentors, mental health, and risk behaviors: A longitudinal analysis of African American adolescents transitioning into adulthood. *Am. J. Community Psychol.* **2010**, *46*, 36–48. [CrossRef]
63. Karcher, M.J. The Study of Mentoring in the Learning Environment (SMILE): A randomized evaluation of the effectiveness of school-based mentoring. *Prev. Sci.* **2008**, *9*, 99–113. [CrossRef]
64. Motti-Stefanidi, F.; Pavlopoulos, V.; Mastrotheodoros, S.; Asendorpf, J. Longitudinal interplay between peer likeability and youth's adaptation and psychological well-being: A study of immigrant and non-immigrant adolescents in the school context. *Int. J. Behav. Dev.* **2020**, *44*, 393–403. [CrossRef]
65. Dalmasso, P.; Borraccino, A.; Lazzeri, G.; Charrier, L.; Berchialla, P.; Cavallo, F.; Lemma, P. Being a young migrant in Italy: The effect of perceived social support in adolescence. *J. Immigr. Minor Health* **2018**, *20*, 1044–1052. [CrossRef]
66. Bernstein, L.; Dun Rappaport, C.; Olsho, L.; Hunt, D.; Levin, M. *Impact Evaluation of the U.S. Department of Education's Student Mentoring Program: Final Report (NCEE 2009-4047)*; U.S. Department of Education, Institute of Education Sciences, National Center for Education Evaluation and Regional Assistance: Washington, DC, USA, 2009.
67. Hurd, N.M.; Sánchez, B.; Zimmerman, M.A.; Caldwell, C.H. Natural mentors, racial identity, and educational attainment among African American adolescents: Exploring pathways to success. *Child Dev.* **2012**, *83*, 1196–1212. [CrossRef]
68. Grossman, J.B.; Rhodes, J.E. The test of time: Predictors and effects of duration in youth mentoring relationships. *Am. J. Community Psychol.* **2002**, *30*, 199–219. [CrossRef] [PubMed]
69. Rhodes, J.E.; Schwartz, S.E.O.; Willis, M.M.; Wu, M.B. Validating a mentoring relationship quality scale: Does match strength predict match length? *Youth Soc.* **2017**, *49*, 415–437. [CrossRef]
70. Dubois, D.L.; Portillo, N.; Rhodes, J.E.; Silverthorn, N.; Valentine, J.C. How Effective are Mentoring Programs for Youth? A Systematic Assessment of the Evidence. *Psychol. Sci. Public Interest* **2011**, *12*, 57–91. [CrossRef] [PubMed]

71. Kanchewa, S.S.; Rhodes, J.E.; Schwartz, S.E.O.; Olsho, L.E.W. An investigation of same-versus cross-gender matching for boys in formal school-based mentoring programs. *Appl. Dev. Sci.* **2014**, *18*, 31–45. [CrossRef]
72. Herrera, C.; Grossman, J.B.; Kauh, T.J.; Feldman, A.F.; McMaken, J. *Making a Difference in Schools. The Big Brothers Big Sisters School-Based Mentoring Impact Study*; Public/Private Ventures: New York, NY, USA, 2007.

Publisher's Note: MDPI stays neutral with regard to jurisdictional claims in published maps and institutional affiliations.

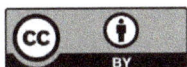

© 2020 by the authors. Licensee MDPI, Basel, Switzerland. This article is an open access article distributed under the terms and conditions of the Creative Commons Attribution (CC BY) license (http://creativecommons.org/licenses/by/4.0/).

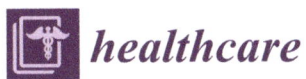

Article

How to Relax in Stressful Situations: A Smart Stress Reduction System

Yekta Said Can [1,*], Heather Iles-Smith [2], Niaz Chalabianloo [1], Deniz Ekiz [1], Javier Fernández-Álvarez [3], Claudia Repetto [3], Giuseppe Riva [3] and Cem Ersoy [1]

1. Computer Engineering Department, Bogazici University, 34342 Istanbul, Turkey; niaz.chalabianloo@boun.edu.tr (N.C.); deniz.ekiz@boun.edu.tr (D.E.); ersoy@boun.edu.tr (C.E.)
2. Leeds Teaching Hospitals NHS Trust/University of Leeds, Leeds LS1 3EX, UK; heather.iles-smith@nhs.net
3. General Psychology and Communication Psychology, Catholic University of Milan, 20123 Milan, Italy; javier.fernandezkirszman@unicatt.it (J.F.-Á.); claudia.repetto@unicatt.it (C.R.); giuseppe.riva@unicatt.it (G.R.)
* Correspondence: yekta.can@boun.edu.tr

Received: 27 February 2020; Accepted: 10 April 2020; Published: 16 April 2020

Abstract: Stress is an inescapable element of the modern age. Instances of untreated stress may lead to a reduction in the individual's health, well-being and socio-economic situation. Stress management application development for wearable smart devices is a growing market. The use of wearable smart devices and biofeedback for individualized real-life stress reduction interventions has received less attention. By using our unobtrusive automatic stress detection system for use with consumer-grade smart bands, we first detected stress levels. When a high stress level is detected, our system suggests the most appropriate relaxation method by analyzing the physical activity-based contextual information. In more restricted contexts, physical activity is lower and mobile relaxation methods might be more appropriate, whereas in free contexts traditional methods might be useful. We further compared traditional and mobile relaxation methods by using our stress level detection system during an eight day EU project training event involving 15 early stage researchers (mean age 28; gender 9 Male, 6 Female). Participants' daily stress levels were monitored and a range of traditional and mobile stress management techniques was applied. On day eight, participants were exposed to a 'stressful' event by being required to give an oral presentation. Insights about the success of both traditional and mobile relaxation methods by using the physiological signals and collected self-reports were provided.

Keywords: commercial smartwatch; mental stress; psychophysiological; emotion regulation; heart rate variability; electrodermal activity

1. Introduction

Stress constitutes a complex process that is activated by a physical or mental threat to the individuals' homeostasis, comprising a set of diverse psychological, physiological and behavioral responses [1]. Although it is usually considered a negative response, stress actually constitutes a key process for ensuring our survival. However, when a stress response is repeatedly triggered in the absence of a challenging stimulus, or if there is constant exposure to challenging situations, stress can become harmful. Evidence suggests that, in either of these two contexts, stress is a persistent factor for the development of psycho-pathological conditions [2,3].

When faced with stressful events, people make autonomic and controlled efforts to reduce the negative impact and maximize the positive impact that every specific situation may provoke. Generally, this process is denominated as emotion regulation, formally defined as the process by which individuals can influence what emotions they have, when they have them and how they experience and express those emotions [4]. It has been suggested that the term emotion regulation can be understood as a broad tag that comprises the regulation of all responses that are emotionally charged, from basic emotions to complex mood states as well as regulation of everyday life [5].

Failure to address triggers of stress has been shown to lead to chronic stress, anxiety and depression, and attributed to serious physical health conditions such as cardiovascular disease [6]. The World Health Organization concluded that psychological stress is one of the most significant health problems in the 21st-century and is a growing problem [7]. There are various interventions to minimize stress based on individual preferences and requirements. Stress management techniques including ancient practices such as Tai Chi [8] and yoga [9] as well as other physical activities [10] are often cited as being helpful in combating stress. Likewise traditional meditation, mindfulness [11] and cognitive behavioural therapy (CBT) [12] all have established benefits. These techniques are not applicable in office or social environments, or during most daily routines. Therefore, a smart device based stress management application may be of benefit. Recently, smartphone applications such as Calm, Pause, Heartmath and Sway have been developed for indoor environments. However, these applications are not individualized nor do they include biofeedback and studies that validate their effects are limited [13].

In this study, we used the stress level detection scheme using physiological signals and added a physical activity based context analyzer. When the user experiences a high stress level, the system suggests appropriate stress reduction methods (traditional or mobile). We further compare the effects of traditional and mobile stress alleviation methods on physiological data of 15 international Ph.D. students (participants) during eight days of training. In addition, 1440 h of physiological signals from Empatica E4 smart bands were collected in this training event. Stress management techniques based on the emotion regulation model of James Gross [4] were applied to reduce participant stress levels. To the best of our knowledge, this work is the first one suggesting appropriate stress reduction methods based on contextual information and comparing both traditional and mobile stress management interventions in the real-life environment using a commercial smart-band based automatic stress level detection system that eliminates motion artifacts. Using such a system is essential because these offline stress level detection algorithms could be used in real-time biofeedback apps.

Application of our stress level detection algorithm, in a real world context, could allow individuals to receive feedback regarding high stress levels along with recommendations for relaxation methods. Additional continued monitoring may also enable the individual to better understand the effectiveness of any stress reduction methods. However, for our stress detection algorithm to be applied in daily life, the smart device should be unobtrusive (i.e., should not be comprised of cables, electrodes, boards). Our system works on smart-bands which are perfect examples of this type of unobtrusive wearable device.

This paper describes emotion regulation in the context of stress management and how yoga and mindfulness can be used for regulating emotions (Section 2). Methods of detecting stress and analyzing context based on physical activity are described (Section 3) and data are presented related to our method for stress level detection with the use of smart-bands (Section 4). Experimental results and discussion are also presented (Section 5) and we present the conclusions and future works of the study (Section 6).

The major research contributions of this study are the following:

- Developing a physical activity based context analyzer and relaxation method suggestion system
- Comparison of stress reduction methods (mobile mindfulness, traditional mindfulness and yoga) and their effectiveness in the context of stress management with the use of an unobtrusive smartwatch based stress level detection system
- Application of James Gross's prominent emotion regulation model in the context of stress management and measuring the physiological component with smart bands.

2. Background

2.1. Emotion Regulation in the Context of Stress Management

Stress is a normal part of daily life. However, its effects often vary across individuals and despite similar circumstances, some people do not feel under strain while others may be severely affected. Multiple reasons exist for these differences between individuals, including how people perceive reality and how they respond to the numerous stimuli to which they are exposed. When a person believes that a certain situation surpasses their available coping mechanisms, it is referred to as perceived stress. Thus, perceived stress varies from person to person depending on the value that an individual gives to a situation and their self-recognition of the resources to deal with it.

Numerous psychological scientists have investigated perceived stress. Individuals who display a mismatch between contextual demands and perceived resources constantly (rather than during a specific moment in time) are referred to as experiencing chronic stress. Chronic stress has not only been shown to be very relevant in people's well-being and quality of life, but also important in the appearance and maintenance of several physical and mental diseases [14].

As a consequence, mounting research has focused on the mechanisms that people implement in order to alleviate the physical and cognitive burden associated with that perceived stress. Coping styles, stress management techniques, self-regulation, or emotion regulation techniques are different labels that define the way people implement certain behavioral, cognitive, or emotional strategies to maintain allosteric load [15]. In other words, every living organism needs to vary among plasticity and stability in order to survive. Human beings are not the exception to the rule and the complex system that applies to every single person and the necessity of reaching a constant level of regulation permits the individuals to pursue their goals.

Specifically, emotion regulation has been defined as the study of "the processes by which we influence which emotions we have when we have them, and how we experience and express them" [4]. A large body of evidence has shown that there are very different consequences depending on the effectiveness people achieve to regulate their emotions. Naturally, both at an implicit or explicit level, people regulate emotions in order to maintain those allosteric levels previously mentioned. Therefore, when there are specific stressors that demand a particular cognitive or physical response, the emotional reactivity may be stronger and the need for a proper regulation more relevant. Indeed, emotion regulation has shown to be a transdiagnostic factor that is present at a wide range of mental disorders. In other words, the way people initiate, implement and monitor their emotional processes, in order to reach more desirable states, has a significant impact on the stress levels. Some emotion regulation (ER) strategies have shown to be correlated with mental health issues. Among these strategies, cognitive reappraisal, problem-solving, or acceptance shall be mentioned as strategies that are negatively correlated with psychopathology, while rumination, experiential avoidance, or suppression are positively correlated with psychopathology [16]. In this regard, hinging on the different ER strategies deployed, ER can constitute a protective factor to face stress responses that all individuals experience after minor or major stressors [17]. Additionally, an adaptive regulation of emotions, by managing stress, may also be beneficial for clinical populations, such as people suffering from affective disorders [18,19].

Therefore, from whole psychotherapeutic treatments to single self-applied applications, studies in the literature have focused on how people can better regulate their emotions and manage their stress levels. Among many other techniques, cognitive behavioral therapy, autogenic training, biofeedback, breathing exercises, relaxation techniques, guided imagery, mindfulness, yoga, or Tai-Chi, are some of the stress management interventions that have received attention from researchers [20,21].

2.2. Yoga and Mindfulness: As Tools for Emotion Regulation

2.2.1. Yoga

Yoga is an ancient Eastern practice that developed more than 2000 years ago. Although its original creator and source are uncertain, the earliest written word 'Yoga Sutra' describes the philosophy of yoga focussing on growing spirituality, regulating emotions and thoughts. Initially, the focus was on awareness of breathing and breathing exercises 'pranayama' to calm the mind and body, ultimately reaching a higher state of consciousness.

As yoga evolved, physical movement in the form of postures was included and integrated with yogic breathing 'prana' and elements of relaxation. The underlying purpose is to create physical flexibility, reduce pain and unpleasant stimuli and reduce negative thoughts and emotions to calm the mind and body, thereby improving well-being. In the healthcare literature, the benefits are reported to be far-reaching both for mental and physical health conditions such as anxiety, depression, cardiovascular disease, cancer and respiratory symptoms. It is also reported to reduce muscular-skeletal problems and physical symptoms through increasing the awareness of the physical body.

Yoga has become a global phenomenon and is widely practiced in many different forms. Generally, all types of yoga include some elements of relaxation. Additionally, some forms include mainly pranayama and others are more physical in nature. One such practice is vinyasa flow which involves using the inhale and exhale of the breathing pattern to move through a variety of yoga postures; this leads to the movement becoming meditative. The practice often includes pranayama followed by standing postures linked together with a movement called vinyasa, (similar to a sun salutation) which helps to keep the body moving and increases fitness, flexibility and helps maintain linkage with the breath. The practice also often includes a range of seated postures, an inversion (such as headstand or shoulder stand) and final relaxation 'savasana'.

2.2.2. Mindfulness

Mindfulness involves being more present at the moment by acknowledging the here and now, often referred to as 'being present' rather than focussing on the past or future [8]. Being present may include being aware of our surroundings and the environment, or of what we are eating and drinking and physical sensations such as the sun or wind on our skin.

Acknowledging the thoughts and body are also aspects of mindfulness. Each day humans experience thousands of thoughts, the majority being of no consequence. In some instances, these thoughts are repetitive and negative in nature which can lead to increased stress and the related unpleasant physical symptoms such as feeling anxious, nausea and tension headaches. Being mindful includes an awareness of our thinking and whether we are caught up with our thoughts rather than being aware of the moment. Additionally, on a daily basis, awareness of the physical body may be minimal; being mindful includes increasing this awareness through becoming more connected with the sensations in the body. This might include experiencing the legs moving when walking, or feeling the ground under the feet or the natural way of the body whilst standing.

Mindfulness has been shown to be of benefit to physical and mental health. It is currently recommended by the National Institute for Clinical Excellence [22] as adjunctive therapy to Cognitive Behavioural Therapy (CBT) for the prevention of relapse depression.

However, it may be challenging for some individuals to do this with a multitude of distractions around them and, therefore, they may choose to identify a particular time and place when and where they can sit in a comfortable position to start to become aware of their breathing and bodily sensations.

2.2.3. Mobile Mindfulness Inspired By Tai-Chi—Pause

Tai-Chi is an internal Chinese martial art practiced for both its defense training, its health benefits and meditation. There is good evidence of benefits for depression, cardiac and stroke rehabilitation and dementia [23]. The term Tai-Chi refers to a philosophy of the forces of yin and yang, related to the moves. An iPhone application Pause inspired by Tai-Chi is used for guided mindfulness which draws upon the principles of mindfulness meditation to trigger the body's rest and digest response, quickly restoring attention [24].

3. Related Work

Researchers have created the ability to detect stress in laboratory environments with medical-grade devices [25–28]; smartwatches and smart bands started to be used for stress level detection studies [29–31]. These devices provide high comfort and rich functionality for the users, but their stress detection accuracies are lower than medical-grade devices due to low signal quality and difficulty obtaining data in intense physical activity. If data are collected for long periods, researchers have shown that their detection performance improves [32]. During movement periods, the signal can be lost (gap in the data) or artifacts might be generated. Stress level detection accuracies for 2-classes by using these devices are around 70% [29,30,33,34].

After detecting the stress level of individuals, researchers should recover from the stressed state to the baseline state. To the best of our knowledge, there are very few studies that combine automatic stress detection (using physiological data) with recommended appropriate stress management techniques. Ahani et al. [35] examined the physiological effect of mindfulness. They used the Biosemi device which acquires electroencephalogram (EEG) and respiration signals. They successfully distinguished control (non-meditative state) and meditation states with machine learning algorithms. Karydis et al. [36] identified the post-meditation perceptual states by using a wearable EEG measurement device (Muse headband). Mason et al. [37] examined the effect of yoga on physiological signals. They used PortaPres Digital Plethtsmograph for measuring blood pressure and respiration signals. They also showed the positive effect of yoga by using these signals. A further study validated the positive effect of yoga with physiological signals; researchers monitored breathing and heart rate pulse with a piezoelectric belt and a pulse sensor [21]. They demonstrated the effectiveness of different yogic breathing patterns to help participants relax. There are also several studies showing the effectiveness of mobile mindfulness apps by using physiological signals [20,38,39]. Svetlov et al. [20] monitored the heart rate variability (HRV), electrodermal activity (EDA), Salivary alpha-amylase (sAA) and EEG values. In other studies, EEG and respiration signals were also used for validating the effect of mobile mindfulness apps [38,39]. When the literature is examined, it could be observed that the effect of ancient relaxation methods and mobile mindfulness methods are examined separately in different studies. Ancient methods generally require out of office environments that are not suitable for most of the population, since, in the modern age, people started to spend more time in office-like environments. On the other hand, some smartphone applications such as Pause, HeartMath and Calm do not require extra hardware or equipment and be applicable in office environments. Hence, an ideal solution depends on the context of individuals. A system that monitors stress levels, analyzes the context of individuals and suggests an appropriate relaxation method in the case of high stress will benefit society. Furthermore, mobile methods along with the ancient techniques should be applied in stressful real-life events and their effectiveness should be compared by investigating physiological signals. When the literature is examined, there is not any study comparing the performance of these methods in real-life events (see Table 1). Another important finding is that these methods should be compared with unobtrusive wearable devices so that they could be used for a biofeedback system in daily lives. Individuals may be reluctant to use a system with cables, electrodes and boards in their daily life. Therefore, a comparison of different states with such systems could not be used in daily life. There is clearly a need for a suggestion and comparison of ancient and mobile meditation methods by using algorithms that could run on unobtrusive devices. An ideal system should detect high stress levels, suggest relaxation methods and control whether users are doing these exercises right or not with unobtrusive devices. Our algorithm is suitable to be embedded in such daily life applicable systems that use physiological signals such as skin temperature (ST), HRV, EDA and accelerometer (ACC). In this paper, we present the findings of our pilot study that tested the use of our algorithm during general daily activities, stress reduction activities and a stressful event.

Table 1. Comparison of our work with the studies applying different types of meditation techniques for stress management in the literature.

Article	YOGA	Mindfulness	Mobile Relaxation	Device	Signal	Daily Suitable
Ahani et al. [35]	X	✓	X	Biosemi	EEG and Respiration	No
Mason et al. [37]	✓	X	X	Digital Plethysmograph (PortaPres)	Virtual Blood Pressure Respiration	No
Svetlov et al. [20]	X	X	✓	Several	HRV, EDA, sAA and EEG	No
Puranik et al. [21]	✓	X	X	MPU 6050 + piezoelectric belt + pulse sensor + smartphone	Heart Rate + Respiration	No
Karydis et al. [36]	X	✓	X	Muse Headband	EEG	No
Cheng et al. [38]	X	X	✓	Emotiv wireless headset	EEG	No
Ingle et al. [39]	X	X	✓	8-channel Enobio EEG + piezoelectric belt	EEG + Respiratory	No
Our work	✓	✓	✓	Empatica E4 wristband	PPG (Photoplethysmography), EDA, ACC, ST	Yes

4. Methodology

4.1. Unobtrusive Stress Detection System with Smart Bands

Our stress detection system developed in [32] allows users to be aware of their stress levels during their daily activities without creating any interruption or restriction. The only requirement to use this system is the need to wear a smart band. Participants in this study wore the Empatica E4 smart band on their non-dominant hand. The smart band provides Blood Volume Pressure, ST, EDA, IBI (Interbeat Interval) and 3D Acceleration. The data are stored in the memory of the device. Then, the artifacts of physiological signals were detected and handled. The features were extracted from the sensory signals and fed to the machine learning algorithm for prediction. In order to use this system, pre-trained machine learning models are required. For training the models, feature vectors and collected class labels were used.

4.1.1. EDA Preprocessing Artifact Detection and Removal Methods

The body sweats when emotional arousal and stress are experienced and, therefore, skin conductance increases [40]. This makes EDA a promising candidate for stress level detection. Intense physical activity and temperature changes contaminate the SC (Skin Conductance) signal. Therefore, affected segments (artifacts) should be filtered out from the original signal. In order to detect the artifacts in the SC signal, we used an EDA toolkit [41] which is 95% accurate on the detection of the artifacts. While developing this tool, technicians labeled the artifacts manually. They trained a machine learning model by using the labels. In addition to the SC signal, 3D acceleration and ST signals were also used for artifact detection. We removed the parts that this tool detected as artifacts from our signals. We further added batch processing and segmentation to this tool by using custom software built-in Python 2.7.

4.1.2. EDA Feature Extraction Methods

After the artifact removal phase, features were extracted from the EDA signal. This signal has two components phasic and tonic; features from both components were extracted (see Table 2). The cvxEDA tool [42] was used for the decomposition of the signal into these components. This tool uses convex optimization to estimate the Autonomic Nervous System (ANS) activity that is based on Bayesian statistics.

Tonic Component Features

The tonic component in the EDA signal represents the long-term slow changes. This component is also known as the skin conductance level. It could be regarded as the indicator of general psychophysiological activation [43].

Table 2. EDA features and their definitions.

Feature	Description
Quartdev Tonic	Quartile deviation (75 percentile–25 percentile) of the phasic component
Strong Peaks Phasic	The number of strong peak per 100 s
Peaks Phasic	The number of peaks per 100 s
Perc20	20th percentile of the phasic component
Perc80 Tonic	80th percentile of the phasic component
Mean Tonic	Mean of the phasic component
SD Tonic	Standard deviation of phasic component

Phasic Component Features

The phasic component represents faster (event-related) differences in the SC signal. The Peaks of phasic SC component as a reaction to a stimulus is also called Skin Conductance Response [43]. After we decompose the phasic component from the EDA signal, peak related features were extracted.

4.1.3. Heart Activity Preprocessing (Artifact Detection and Removal) and Feature Extraction Methods

Heart activity (or, more specifically, HRV) reacts to changes in the autonomic nervous system (ANS) caused by stress [44] and it is, therefore, one of the most commonly used physiological signal for stress detection [40]. However, vigorous movement of subjects and improperly worn devices may contaminate the HRV signal collected from smartwatches and smart bands. In order to address this issue, we developed an artifact handling tool in MATLAB programming language [45] that has batch processing capability. First, the data were divided into 2 min long segments with 50% overlapping. Two-minute segments were selected because it is reported that the time interval for stress stimulation and recovery processes is around a few minutes [46]. The artifact detection percentage rule (also employed in Kubios [47]) was applied after the segmentation phase. In this rule, each data point was compared with the local average around it. When the difference was more than a predetermined threshold percentage, (20% is commonly selected in the literature [48]), the data point was labeled as an artifact. In our system, we deleted the inter-beat intervals detected as the artifacts and interpolated these points with the cubic spline interpolation technique which was used in the Kubios software [47]. The time-domain features of HRV are calculated. In order to calculate the frequency domain features, we interpolated the RR intervals to 4 Hz. Then, we applied the Fast Fourier Transform (FFT). These time and frequency domain features (see Table 3) were selected because these are the most discriminative ones in the literature [30,49,50].

Table 3. HRV features and their definitions [32].

Feature	Description
Mean RR	Mean value of the inter-beat (RR) intervals
STD RR	Standard deviation of the inter-beat interval
pNN50	Percentage of the number of successive RR intervals varying more than 50 ms from the previous interval
RMSSD	Root mean square of successive difference of the RR intervals
SDSD	Related standard deviation of successive RR interval differences
HRV triangular index	Total number of RR intervals divided by the height of the histogram of all RR intervals measured on a scale with bins of 1/128 s
TINN	Triangular interpolation of RR interval histogram
LF	Power in low-frequency band (0.04–0.15 Hz)
HF	Power in high-frequency band (0.15–0.4 Hz)
pLF	Prevalent low-frequency oscillation of heart rate
pHF	Prevalent high-frequency oscillation of heart rate
VLF	Power in very low-frequency band (0.00–0.04 Hz)
LF/HF	Ratio of LF-to-HF

4.1.4. Accelerometer Feature Extraction Methods

Research has shown that movements of the human body and postures can indeed be employed as a means to detect signs of different emotional states. The dynamics of body movement were investigated by Castellano et al. who used multimodal data to identify human affective behaviors. Specific movement metrics, such as the amount of movement, intensity and fluidity, were used to help deduct emotions, and it was found that the amount of movement was a major factor in distinguishing different types of emotions [51]. Melzer et al. investigated whether movements comprised of collections of Laban movement components could be recognized as expressing basic emotions [52]. The results of their study confirm that, even when the subject has no intention of expressing emotions, particular movements can assist in the perception of bodily expressions of emotions. Accelerometer sensors may be used to detect these movements and different types of affect. The accelerometer sensor data are used for two different purposes in our system. Firstly, we extracted features from the accelerometer sensor, for detecting stress levels. We also selected the features to be used as described in Table 4 [53] and, as mentioned above, this sensor was also employed to clean the EDA signal in the EDAExplorer Tool [41].

Table 4. ACC features and their definitions.

Feature	Description
Mean X	Mean acceleration over x axis
Mean Y	Mean acceleration over y axis
Mean Z	Mean acceleration over z axis
MeanAccMag	Mean acceleration over acceleration magnitude
Energy	FFT energy over mean acceleration magnitude

4.1.5. Skin Temperature

A skin temperature signal is used for the artifact detection phase of the EDA signal in the EDAExplorer Tool [41]. After we divide our data into segments, different modalities were merged into one feature vector. The heart activity signal started with a delay (to calculate heartbeats per minute at the start) and all signals were then synchronized. We included start and end timestamps for each segment, and each modality was merged with a custom Python script.

4.1.6. Machine Learning Classifier Algorithms

The Weka machine learning toolkit [54] is used for identifying stress levels. The Weka toolkit has several preprocessing features before classification. Our data set was not balanced when the number of instances belonging to each class was considered. We solved this issue by removing samples from the majority class. We selected random undersampling because it is the most commonly applied method [55]. In this way, we prevented classifiers from biasing towards the class with more instances. In this study, we employed five different machine learning classification algorithms to recognize different stress levels: MultiLayer Perceptron (MLP), Random Forest (RF) (with 100 trees), K-nearest neighbors (kNN) (n = 1–4), Linear discriminant analysis (LDA), Principal component analysis (PCA) and support vector machine (SVM) with a radial basis function. These algorithms were selected because they were the most commonly applied and successful classifiers for detecting stress levels [30,48]. In addition, 10-fold stratified cross-validation was then applied and hyperparameters of the machine learning algorithms were fine-tuned with grid search. The best performing models have been reported.

4.1.7. Dimensionality Reduction

We applied correlation-based feature selection (CBFS) technique which is available in the Weka machine learning package for combined signal [56]. The CBFS method removes the features that are less correlated with the output class. For every model, we selected the ten most important features. This method is applied for MLP, RF, kNN and LDA. In order to create an SVM based model, we applied PCA based dimensionality reduction where the covered variance is selected as 0.95 (the default setting).

4.1.8. Insights from the Feature Selection Process

The CBFS method computes the correlation of features with the ground truth label of the stress level. Insights about the contribution of the features to the stress detection performance can be obtained from Figures 1 and 2. Three of the best features (over 0.15 correlation) are frequency domain features. These features are high, low and very-low frequency components of the HRV signal (see Figure 1). When we examine the EDA features, peaks per 100 s feature is the most important and distinctive feature by far. Since the EDA signal is distorted under the influence of the stimuli, the number of peaks and valleys increases. Lastly, when the acceleration signal is investigated, the most discriminative feature is mean acceleration in the z-axis (see Figure 2b). This could be due to the nature of hand and body gestures which are caused by stressed situations.

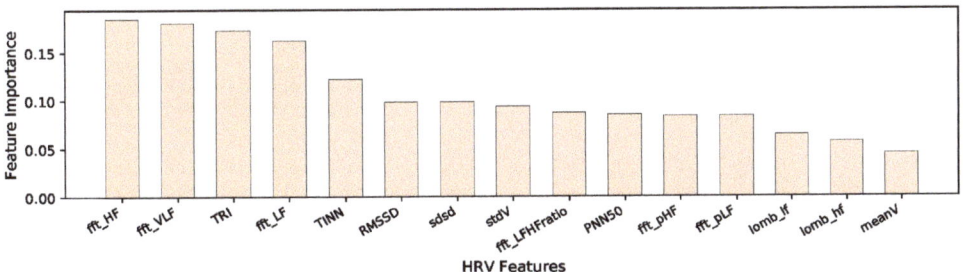

Figure 1. Top-ranking features selected for the HRV signal.

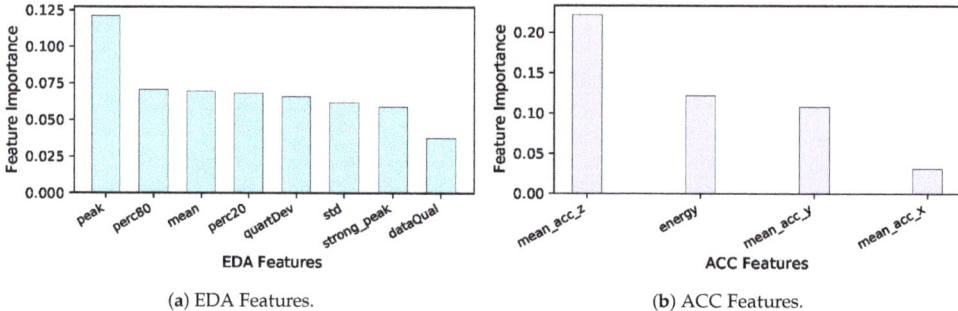

(a) EDA Features. (b) ACC Features.

Figure 2. Top-ranking features selected for the EDA and ACC signals.

4.2. Relaxation Method Suggestion by Analyzing the Physical Activity-Based Context

Context is a broad term that could contain different types of information such as calendars, activity type, location and activity intensity. Physical activity intensity could be used to infer contextual information. In more restricted environments such as office, classrooms, public transportation and physical activity intensity could be low, whereas, in outdoor environments, physical activity intensity could increase. Therefore, an appropriate relaxation method will change according to the context of individuals.

For calculating physical activity intensity, we used the EDAExplorer tool [41]. The stillness metric is used for this purpose. It is the percentage of periods in which the person is still or motionless. Total acceleration must be less than a threshold (default is 0.1 [41]) for 95 percent of a minute in order for this minute to count as still [41]. Then, the ratio of still minutes in a session can be calculated. For the ratio of still minutes in a session, we labeled sessions below 20% as still, above 20% as active and suggested relaxation method accordingly (see Figure 3).

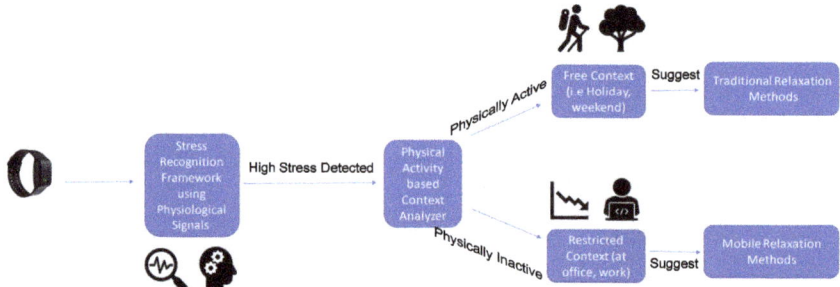

Figure 3. The whole system diagram is depicted. When a high stress level is experienced, by analyzing the physical activity based context, the system suggests the most appropriate reduction method.

4.3. Description of the Data Collection Procedure

The proposed stress level monitoring mechanism, for real-life settings, was evaluated during an eight day Marie Skłodowska-Curie Innovative Training Network (ITN) training event in Istanbul, Turkey, for the AffecTech project. AffecTech is a program funded by Horizon 2020 (H2020) framework established by the European Commission. The AffecTech project is an international collaborative research network involving 15 PhD students (early stage researchers (ESR)) with the aim of developing low-cost effective wearable technologies for individuals who experience affective disorders (for example, depression, anxiety and bipolar disorder).

The eight-day training event included workshops, lectures and training with clearly defined tasks and activities to ensure that the ESR had developed the required skills, knowledge and values outline prior to the training event. At the end of the eight-day training, ESRs were required to deliver a presentation about their PhD work to two evaluators from the European Union where they received feedback about their progress (see Figure 4 for raw physiological signals at the start of the presentation). For studying the effects of emotion regulation on stress, yoga, guided mindfulness and mobile-based mindfulness, sessions were held by a certified instructor.

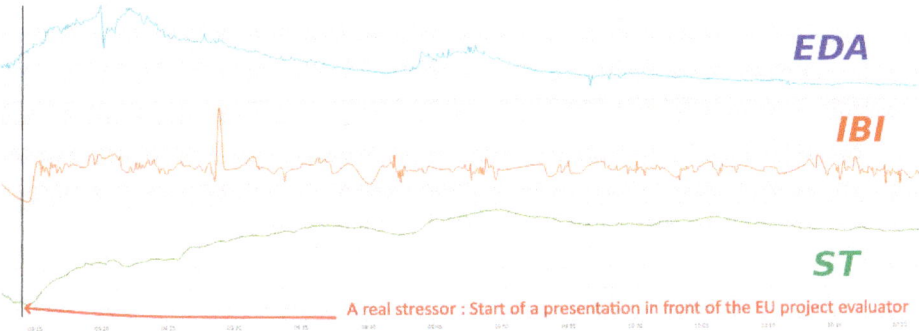

Figure 4. Sample data belong to a presentation session. The increase in EDA, ST and IBI could be observed when the subject started the presentation.

During the training, physiological and questionnaire data were collected from the 16 ESR participants (9 men, mean age 28); 15 ESRs and one of the AffecTech project academics, all of whom gave informed consent to participate in the study. Participants were from different countries with diverse nationalities (two from Iran, two from Spain, two from Italy, one from Argentina, one from Pakistan, one from China, one from Switzerland, one from Belarus, one from France, one from England, one from Barbados, one from Turkey and one from Bulgaria). Due to the fault of one of the Empatica E4 devices, it was not possible to include data from one participant. The remaining 15 participants completed all stages of the study successfully.

During the eight days of training and presentations, psychophysiological data were collected from 16 participants during the training event from Empatica E4 smart band while they are awake. For studying the effects of emotion regulation on stress, yoga, guided mindfulness and mobile-based mindfulness sessions were held by a certified instructor. The timeline of the event is shown in Figure 5.

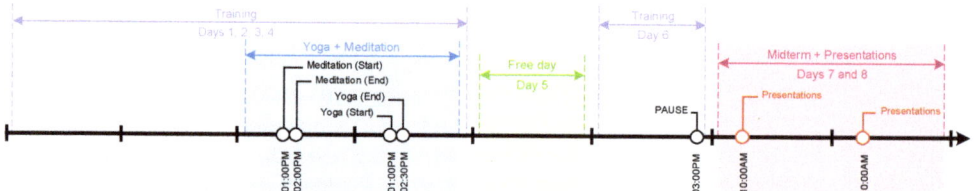

Figure 5. Time-line depicting eight days of the training event. Presentations, relaxations and lectures are highlighted.

4.3.1. Physiological Stress Data

The psychophysiological signal data were collected using the Empatica E4 smart band whilst participants were awake throughout the eight days of the AffecTech training. Physiological data included IBI, EDA, ACC (Accelerometer) and ST and stored in different csv files. In addition, 27.39% of the data are obtained from free times (free day and after training until subjects slept 5:00 p.m.–10:00 p.m.), 43.83% of the data comes from lectures in the training, 11.41% is the presentation session and relax sessions consist of 17.35% of the data. As mentioned previously, we randomly undersampled (most commonly applied method [55]) the data to overcome the class imbalance problem. The participants' blood pressure (BP) was also recorded using CE(0123) Harvard Medical Devices Ltd. automated sphygmomanometer prior to and after each stress reduction event (yoga and mindfulness), in order to demonstrate whether the participants stress levels were modified. On each occasion that the participants' BP was recorded, the mean of three recordings was used as the final BP. A reduction in the participants' blood pressure and/or pulse rate may be seen, which demonstrates a reduction in stress level.

4.3.2. Ethics

The procedure used in this study was approved by the Institutional Review Board for Research with Human Subjects of Boğaziçi University with the approval number 2018/16. Prior to data acquisition, each participant received a consent form describing the experimental procedure and its benefits and implications to both the society and the subject. The procedure was also explained verbally to the subject. All of the data are stored anonymously.

4.3.3. Questionnaire Self-Report Stress Data

A session-based self-report questionnaire comprised of six questions based on the Nasa Task Load Index (NASA-TLX) [57]. The frustration scale was specifically used to measure perceived stress levels [32]. We asked the following question to the participants for each session:

How irritated, stressed and annoyed versus content, relaxed and complacent did you feel during the task?

Questionnaires were completed daily (at the end of the day) and, after each presentation, lecture and stress reduction event (such as yoga and mindfulness).

4.3.4. Stress Management Scheme Using Yoga and Mindfulness

During the eight day training, it is assumed that the participants' stress levels are likely to have increased day by day because they were required to give a presentation (perceived as a stressful event) reporting their PhD progress to the EU project evaluators at the end of the training.

Underpinned by James Gross's Emotion Regulation model (see Figure 6) [4], we modified the situation to help the participants to reduce their thoughts of the end of the training presentation. To help participants manage their stress levels, we applied Yoga and mindfulness sessions on two separate days (day three and day four, respectively). These sessions lasted approximately 1 h and, throughout the sessions, participants wore an Empatica E4 smartband. In addition to the physiological signals coming from the Smartbands, participants' blood pressure values were also recorded before and after the yoga and mindfulness sessions.

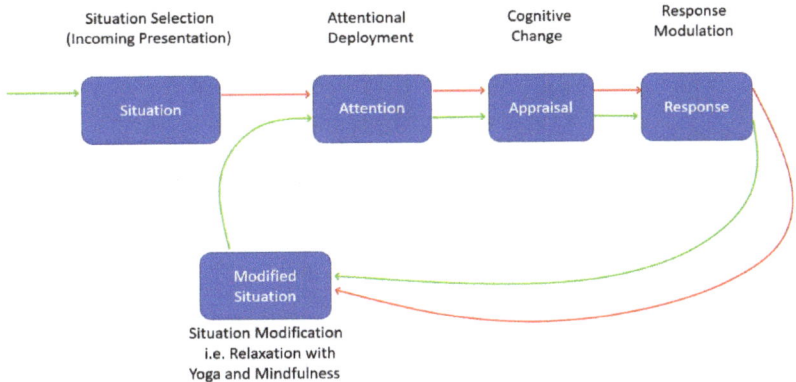

Figure 6. Application of James Gross's Emotion Regulation model [4] in the context of stress management.

5. Experimental Results and Discussion

5.1. Statistical Data Analysis

5.1.1. Validation of Different Perceived Stress Levels by using the Self-Reports

In order to validate that the participants experienced different perceived stress levels in different contexts (lecture, relaxation, presentation), we used the Frustration item (see Section 4.5) from the NASA-TLX [57]. The distribution of answers is demonstrated in Figure 7. Our aim is to show that the perceived stress levels (obtained from self-report answers) differ in relaxation sessions considerably when compared to the presentation session (high stress). To this end, we applied the t-test (in R programming language) to the perceived stress self-report answers of yoga versus presentation, mindfulness versus presentation and pause (mobile mindfulness) versus presentation session pairs. The paired t-test is used to evaluate the separability of each session. The degree of freedom is 15. We applied the variance test to each session tuple; we could not identify equal variance in any of the session tuples. Thus, we selected the variance as unequal. We used 99.5% confidence intervals. The t-test results' (p-values and test statistics) are provided in Table 5. For all tuples, the null hypothesis stating that the perceived stress of the relaxation method is not less than the presentation session is rejected. The perceived stress levels of participants for all meditation sessions are observed to be significantly lower than the presentation session (high stress).

Table 5. T-test results for session tuple comparison of perceived stress levels using self-reports.

Session Tuple	t-Test Statistic	p-Value
Yoga—Presentation	−4.0027	$p < 0.005$
Guided Mindfulness—Presentation	−5.4905	$p < 0.005$
Mobile Mindfulness—Presentation	−4.2677	$p < 0.005$

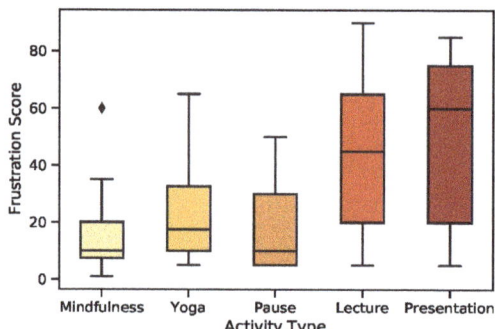

Figure 7. Visual representation of the frustration scores collected in different types of sessions.

5.1.2. Before and After Physiological Measurements for Evaluating Performance of Yoga and Mindfulness with Blood Pressure

In this section, we compared the effect of stress management tools such as yoga and mindfulness on blood pressure. It is expected that blood pressure sensors will be part of unobtrusive wrist-worn wearable sensors soon. We plan to integrate a blood pressure (BP) module to our system when they are available. Therefore, by using the measurements of a medical-grade blood pressure monitor, we provided insights about how stress reaction affects BP. We further applied and tested the prominent emotion regulation model of James Gross by analyzing these measurements in the context of stress management. We measured the diastolic and systolic BP and pulse using a medical-grade blood pressure monitor before and after the yoga and mindfulness sessions. In order to ensure that the participants were relaxed and that an accurate BP was recorded, BP was measured three times with the mean as the recorded result. A one-sample t-test was applied to the difference between mean values. The results are shown in Table 6.

Mindfulness decreased the systolic BP, -1.13% (ns), increased diastolic BP, $+1.75\%$ ($p < 0.05$) and decreased the pulse -5.75% ($p < 0.05$). Medicine knows that systolic blood pressure (the top number or highest blood pressure when the heart is squeezing and pushing the blood around the body) is more important than diastolic blood pressure (the bottom number or lowest blood pressure between heartbeats) because it gives the best idea of the risk of having a stroke or heart attack. In this view, the significant reduction of systolic BP after mindfulness is an important result.

Moreover, the difference between systolic and diastolic BP is called pulse pressure. For example, 120 systolic minus 60 diastolic equals a pulse pressure of 60. It is also known that a pulse pressure greater than 60 can be a predictor of heart attacks or other cardiovascular diseases, while a low pulse pressure (less than 40) may indicate poor heart function. In our study, pulse pressure was lower after mindfulness (we had both a significant reduction in systolic BP and an increase in diastolic BP), but its value was higher than 40 (42.69 mean difference before the mindfulness and 40.48 mean difference after the mindfulness), suggesting that this result can also be considered clinically positive.

During yoga, there was a decrease in systolic BP by -5.81% ($p < 0.05$), diastolic BP by -1.93% (ns) and increase in pulse $+8.06\%$ ($p < 0.05$). Yoga appears to be more effective than mindfulness at decreasing systolic and diastolic blood pressure, although mindfulness seems to be more effective than yoga for decreasing the pulse due to the activity involved in yoga.

Table 6. The difference between the mean diastolic blood pressure, the mean systolic blood pressure and the mean pulse, before and after sessions of guided mindfulness and guided yoga. (* $p < 0.05$).

Activity	Systolic	Diastolic	Pulse
Guided Mindfulness	−1.31%	1.75% *	−5.75% *
Guided Yoga	−5.81% *	−1.93%	8.06% *

5.2. Physiological Stress Level Detection with Wearables by Using Context Labels as the Class Label

We tested our system by using the known context labels of sessions as the class label. We used Lecture (mild stress), Yoga and Mindfulness (relax) and Presentation in front of the board of juries (high stress) as class labels by examining perceived stress self-report answers in Figure 6. We investigated the success of relaxation methods, different modalities and finding the presenter.

5.2.1. Effect of Different Physiological Signals on Stress Detection

We evaluated the effect of using the interbeat-interval, the skin conductance and the accelerometer signals separately and in a combined manner on two and three class classification performance. These classes are mild stress, high stress and relax states from mindfulness and yoga sessions. The results are shown in Tables 7–9. For the three-class classification problem, we achieved a maximum accuracy of 72% by using MLP on only HRV features and 86.61% with only accelerometer features using the Random Forest classifier and 85.36% accuracy combination of all features with LDA classifier (see Table 7). The difficulty in this classification task is a similar physiological reaction to relax and mild stress situations. However, since the main focus of our study is to discriminate high stress from other classes to offer relaxation techniques in this state, it did not affect our system performance. We also investigated high-mild stress and high stress-relax 2-class classification performance. For the discrimination of high and mild stress, HRV outperformed other signals with 98% accuracy using MLP (see Table 8). In the high stress-relax 2-class problem, only HRV features with RF achieved a maximum accuracy of 86%, whereas ACC features with MLP achieved a maximum of 94% accuracy. In this problem, the combination of all signals with RF achieved 92% accuracy which is the best among all classifiers (see Table 9). For all models, EDA did not perform well. This might be caused by the loose contact with EDA electrodes in the strap due to loosely worn smartbands.

Table 7. Effect of different modalities and their combination on the system performance. Note that the number of classes is fixed at 3 (high stress, mild stress and relax).

Algorithm	Accuracy, %			
	HRV	EDA	ACC	Combined
MLP	72.14	36.61	74.29	82.68
RF	67.86	36.96	86.61	85.18
kNN	65.00	29.82	70.89	78.39
LDA	69.82	31.96	73.39	85.36
SVM	47.14	30.54	58.57	46.96

Table 8. Effect of different modalities and their combination on the system performance. Note that the number of classes is fixed at 2 (high stress and mild stress).

Algorithm	Accuracy, %			
	HRV	EDA	ACC	Combined
MLP	98.00	60.00	64.00	98.00
RF	98.00	42.00	72.00	98.00
kNN	94.00	44.00	58.00	94.00
LDA	94.00	40.00	54.00	94.00
SVM	66.00	54.00	54.00	66.00

Table 9. Effect of different modalities and their combination on the system performance. Note that the number of classes is fixed at 2 (high stress and relax).

Algorithm	Accuracy, %			
	HRV	EDA	ACC	Combined
MLP	82.00	66.00	96.00	90.00
RF	86.00	60.00	94.00	92.00
kNN	82.00	66.00	88.00	90.00
LDA	78.00	64.00	92.00	88.00
SVM	78.00	62.00	52.00	74.00

5.2.2. Effectiveness of Yoga, Mindfulness and Mobile Mindfulness (Pause)

We applied three different relaxation methods to manage stress levels of individuals. In order to measure the effectiveness of each method, we examined how easily these physiological signals in the relaxation sessions can be separated from high stress presentations. If it can be separated from high stress levels with higher classification performance, it could be inferred that they are more successful at reducing stress. As seen in Tables 10 and 11, mobile mindfulness has lower success in reducing stress levels. Yoga has the highest classification performance with both HR and EDA signals.

Table 10. The classification accuracy of the relaxation sessions using stress management methods and stressful sessions using EDA.

Algorithm	Accuracy, %		
	Guided Mindfulness	Yoga	Mobile Mindfulness
MLP	65.71	78.57	75.00
RF	67.14	87.14	67.64
kNN	64.29	82.86	77.94
LDA	65.71	80.00	51.47
SVM	70.00	72.86	58.82

Table 11. The classification accuracy of the relaxation sessions using stress management methods and stressful sessions using HRV.

Algorithm	Accuracy, %		
	Guided Mindfulness	Yoga	Mobile Mindfulness
MLP	90.00	97.50	93.94
RF	97.50	95.00	87.89
kNN	90.00	90.00	93.93
LDA	87.50	87.50	75.75
SVM	85.00	80.00	81.82

6. Conclusions

In this study, by using our automatic stress detection system with the use of Empatica-E4 smart-bands, we detected stress levels and suggested appropriate relaxation methods (i.e., traditional or mobile) when high stress levels are experienced. Our stress detection framework is unobtrusive, comfortable and suitable for use in daily life and our relaxation method suggestion system makes its decisions based on the physical activity-related context of a user. To test our system, we collected eight days of data from 16 individuals participating in an EU research project training event. Individuals were exposed to varied stressful and relaxation events (1) training and lectures (mild stress), (2) yoga, mindfulness and mobile mindfulness (PAUSE) (relax) and (3) were required to give a moderated presentation (high stress). The participants were from different countries with diverse cultures.

In addition, 1440 h of mobile data (12 h in a day) were collected during this eight-day event from each participant measuring their stress levels. Data were collected during the training sessions, relaxation events and the moderated presentation and during their free time for 12 h in a day, demonstrating that our study monitored daily life stress. EDA and HR signals were collected to detect physiological stress and a combination of different modalities increased stress detection, performance and provided the most discriminative features. We first applied James Gross ER model in the context of stress management and measured the blood pressure during the ER cycle. When the known context was used as the label for stress level detection system, we achieved 98% accuracy for 2-class and 85% accuracy for 3-class. Most of the studies in the literature only detect stress levels of individuals. The participants' stress levels were managed with yoga, mindfulness and a mobile mindfulness application while monitoring their stress levels. We investigated the success of each stress management technique by the separability of physiological signals from high-stress sessions. We demonstrated that yoga and traditional mindfulness performed slightly better than the mobile mindfulness application. Furthermore, this study is not without limitations. In order to generalize the conclusions, more experiments based on larger sample groups should be conducted. As future work, we plan to develop personalized perceived stress models by using self-reports and test our system in the wild. Furthermore, attitudes in the psychological field constitute a topic of utmost relevance, which always play an instrumental role in the determination of human behavior [58]. We plan to design a new experiment which accounts for the attitudes of participants towards relaxation methods and their effects on the performance of stress recognition systems.

Author Contributions: Y.S.C. is the main editor of this work and made major contributions in data collection, analysis and manuscript writing. H.I.-S. made valuable contributions in both data collection and manuscript writing. She was the yoga and mindfulness instructor in the event and contributed the related sections regarding traditional and mobile methods. She also led the blood pressure measurement efforts before and after relaxation methods. D.E. and N.C. contributed equally to this work in design, implementation, data analysis and writing the manuscript. J.F.-Á., C.R. and G.R. contributed the experiment design and provided valuable insights into both emotion regulation theory. They also contributed to the related sections in the manuscript. C.E. provided invaluable feedback and technical guidance to interpret the design and the detail of the field study. He also performed comprehensive critical editing to increase the overall quality of the manuscript. All authors have read and agreed to the published version of the manuscript.

Funding: This work has been supported by AffecTech: Personal Technologies for Affective Health, Innovative Training Network funded by the H2020 People Programme under Marie Skłodowska-Curie Grant Agreement No. 722022. This work is supported by the Turkish Directorate of Strategy and Budget under the TAM Project number DPT2007K120610.

Acknowledgments: We would like to show our gratitude to the Affectech Project for providing us the opportunity for the data collection in the training event and funding the research.

Conflicts of Interest: The authors declare no conflict of interest.

References

1. Bali, A.; Jaggi, A.S. Clinical experimental stress studies: Methods and assessment. *Rev. Neurosci.* **2015**, *26*, 555–579. [CrossRef] [PubMed]
2. Ingram, R.E.; Luxton, D.D. Vulnerability-stress models. In *Development of Psychopathology: A Vulnerability-Stress Perspective*; SAGE Publications: Thousand Oaks, CA, USA, 2005; pp. 32–46.
3. Harkness, K.L.; Hayden, E.P. *The Oxford Handbook of Stress and Mental Health*; Oxford University Press: Oxford, UK, 2018.
4. Gross, J.J. The emerging field of emotion regulation: An integrative review. *Rev. Gen. Psychol.* **1998**, *2*, 271–299. [CrossRef]
5. Koole, S.L.; Aldao, A. The self-regulation of emotion: Theoretical and empirical advances. In *Handbook of Self-Regulation: Research, Theory and Applications*; Guilford Publications: New York, NY, USA, 2016; pp. 24–41.
6. Dimsdale, J.E. Psychological Stress and Cardiovascular Disease. *J. Am. Coll. Cardiol.* **2008**, *51*, 1237–1246. [CrossRef] [PubMed]
7. Fink, G. Stress: Concepts, Definition and History. 2017. Fink, G. Stress: Definition and history. In *Stress Science: Neuroendocrinology*; Elsevier Publishing: Amsterdam, The Netherlands, 2010; pp. 3–9.
8. Exercise: A Guide to Tai Chi. 2019. Available online: https://www.nhs.uk/live-well/exercise/guide-to-tai-chi (accessed on 25 February 2020).
9. Chong, C.S.; Tsunaka, M.; Chan, E.P. Effects of yoga on stress management in healthy adults: A systematic review. *Altern. Ther. Health Med.* **2011**, *17*, 32.
10. Asmundson, G.J.; Fetzner, M.G.; DeBoer, L.B.; Powers, M.B.; Otto, M.W.; Smits, J.A. Let's get physical: A contemporary review of the anxiolytic effects of exercise for anxiety and its disorders. *Depress. Anxiety* **2013**, *30*, 362–373. [CrossRef]
11. Song, Y.; Lindquist, R. Effects of mindfulness-based stress reduction on depression, anxiety, stress and mindfulness in Korean nursing students. *Nurse Educ. Today* **2015**, *35*, 86–90. [CrossRef]
12. Arch, J.J.; Ayers, C.R.; Baker, A.; Almklov, E.; Dean, D.J.; Craske, M.G. Randomized clinical trial of adapted mindfulness-based stress reduction versus group cognitive behavioral therapy for heterogeneous anxiety disorders. *Behav. Res. Ther.* **2013**, *51*, 185–196. [CrossRef]
13. Cheng, P.; Lucero, A.; Buur, J. PAUSE: Exploring Mindful Touch Interaction on Smartphones. In Proceedings of the 20th International Academic Mindtrek Conference (AcademicMindtrek'16), Tampere, Finland, 17–18 October 2016; ACM: New York, NY, USA, 2016; pp. 184–191.
14. Harkness, K.; Hayden, E.; Olino, T.; Mennies, R.; Wojcieszak, Z. Personality-Stress Vulnerability Models. In *The Oxford Handbook of Stress and Mental Health*; Oxford University Press: Oxford, UK, 2020.
15. McEwen, B.S. Stressed or stressed out: What is the difference? *J. Psychiatry Neurosci.* **2005**, *30*, 315.
16. Aldao, A.; Nolen-Hoeksema, S. The influence of context on the implementation of adaptive emotion regulation strategies. *Behav. Res. Ther.* **2012**, *50*, 493–501. [CrossRef]
17. Troy, A.S.; Mauss, I.B. Resilience in the face of stress: Emotion regulation as a protective factor. *Resil. Ment. Heal. Chall. Across Lifesp.* **2011**, *1*, 30–44.

18. Mennin, D.S.; Fresco, D.M.; Ritter, M.; Heimberg, R.G. An open trial of emotion regulation therapy for generalized anxiety disorder and cooccurring depression. *Depress. Anxiety* **2015**, *32*, 614–623. [CrossRef] [PubMed]
19. Radkovsky, A.; McArdle, J.J.; Bockting, C.L.H.; Berking, M. Successful emotion regulation skills application predicts subsequent reduction of symptom severity during treatment of major depressive disorder. *J. Consult. Clin. Psychol.* **2014**, *82*, 248–262. [CrossRef] [PubMed]
20. Svetlov, A.S.; Nelson, M.M.; Antonenko, P.D.; McNamara, J.P.; Bussing, R. Commercial mindfulness aid does not aid short-term stress reduction compared to unassisted relaxation. *Heliyon* **2019**, *5*, e01351. [CrossRef] [PubMed]
21. Puranik, K.A.; M, K. Wearable Device for Yogic Breathing. In Proceedings of the 2019 Amity International Conference on Artificial Intelligence (AICAI), Dubai, UAE, 4–6 February 2019; pp. 605–610.
22. NICE. *Depression in Adults: Recognition and Management. Clinical Guideline [CG90]*; National Institute for Clinical Excellence: London, UK, 2009.
23. Huston, P.; McFarlane, B. Health benefits of tai chi. *Can. Fam. Physician* **2016**, *62*, 881–890.
24. PauseAble—Mindfulness in Motion. Available online: https://www.pauseable.com/ (accessed on 24 November 2019).
25. Castaldo, R.; Montesinos, L.; Melillo, P.; Massaro, S.; Pecchia, L. To What Extent Can We Shorten HRV Analysis in Wearable Sensing? A Case Study on Mental Stress Detection. In *EMBEC & NBC 2017*; Springer: Singapore, 2018; pp. 643–646.
26. Fernández, J.R.M.; Anishchenko, L. Mental stress detection using bioradar respiratory signals. *Biomed. Signal Process. Control* **2018**, *43*, 244–249. [CrossRef]
27. Giannakakis, G.; Pediaditis, M.; Manousos, D.; Kazantzaki, E.; Chiarugi, F.; Simos, P.G.; Marias, K.; Tsiknakis, M. Stress and anxiety detection using facial cues from videos. *Biomed. Signal Process. Control* **2017**, *31*, 89–101. [CrossRef]

28. Castaldo, R.; Xu, W.; Melillo, P.; Pecchia, L.; Santamaria, L.; James, C. Detection of mental stress due to oral academic examination via ultra-short-term HRV analysis. In Proceedings of the 2016 38th Annual International Conference of the IEEE Engineering in Medicine and Biology Society (EMBC), Orlando, FL, USA, 16–20 August 2016; pp. 3805–3808.
29. Vildjiounaite, E.; Kallio, J.; Kyllönen, V.; Nieminen, M.; Mäntyjärvi, J.; Gimel'farb, G. Unobtrusive stress detection on the basis of smartphone usage data. *Pers. Ubiquitous Comput.* **2018**, doi:10.1007/s00779-017-1108-z. [CrossRef]
30. Gjoreski, M.; Luštrek, M.; Gams, M.; Gjoreski, H. Monitoring stress with a wrist device using context. *J. Biomed. Inform.* **2017**, *73*, 159–170. [CrossRef]
31. Gjoreski, M.; Gjoreski, H.; Luštrek, M.; Gams, M. Continuous Stress Detection Using a Wrist Device: In Laboratory and Real Life. In Proceedings of the 2016 ACM International Joint Conference on Pervasive and Ubiquitous Computing: Adjunct (UbiComp'16), Heidelberg, Germany, 12–16 September 2016; ACM: New York, NY, USA, 2016; pp. 1185–1193.
32. Can, Y.S.; Chalabianloo, N.; Ekiz, D.; Ersoy, C. Continuous Stress Detection Using Wearable Sensors in Real Life: Algorithmic Programming Contest Case Study. *Sensors* **2019**, *19*, 1849. [CrossRef]
33. Ciman, M.; Wac, K. Individuals' stress assessment using human-smartphone interaction analysis. *IEEE Trans. Affect. Comput.* **2016**, *9*, 51–65. [CrossRef]
34. Sysoev, M.; Kos, A.; PogaǎžNik, M. Noninvasive Stress Recognition Considering the Current Activity. *Pers. Ubiquitous Comput.* **2015**, *19*, 1045–1052. [CrossRef]
35. Ahani, A.; Wahbeh, H.; Miller, M.; Nezamfar, H.; Erdogmus, D.; Oken, B. Change in physiological signals during mindfulness meditation. In Proceedings of the 2013 6th International IEEE/EMBS Conference on Neural Engineering (NER), San Diego, CA, USA, 6–8 November 2013; pp. 1378–1381.
36. Karydis, T.; Langer, S.; Foster, S.L.; Mershin, A. Identification of Post-meditation Perceptual States Using Wearable EEG and Self-Calibrating Protocols. In Proceedings of the 11th PErvasive Technologies Related to Assistive Environments Conference (PETRA'18), Corfu, Greece, 26–29 June 2018; ACM: New York, NY, USA, 2018; pp. 566–569; doi:10.1145/3197768.3201544. [CrossRef]
37. Mason, H.; Vandoni, M.; Debarbieri, G.; Codrons, E.; Ugargol, V.; Bernardi, L. Cardiovascular and respiratory effect of yogic slow breathing in the yoga beginner: What is the best approach? *Evid.-Based Complement. Altern. Med.* **2013**, *2013*, 743504. [CrossRef]
38. Pause EEG Validation Article. Available online: https://www.ustwo.com/blog/the-story-of-pause (accessed on 24 November 2019).
39. Ingle, R.; Awale, R. Impact Analysis of Meditation on Physiological Signals. *JOIV Int. J. Inform. Vis.* **2018**, *2*, 31–36. [CrossRef]
40. Can, Y.S.; Arnrich, B.; Ersoy, C. Stress Detection in Daily Life Scenarios Using Smart Phones and Wearable Sensors: A Survey. *J. Biomed. Inform.* **2019**, *92*, 103139. [CrossRef]
41. Taylor, S.; Jaques, N.; Chen, W.; Fedor, S.; Sano, A.; Picard, R. Automatic identification of artifacts in electrodermal activity data. In Proceedings of the 2015 37th Annual International Conference of the IEEE Engineering in Medicine and Biology Society (EMBC), Milan, Italy, 25–29 August 2015; pp. 1934–1937.
42. Greco, A.; Valenza, G.; Lanata, A.; Scilingo, E.P.; Citi, L. cvxEDA: A Convex Optimization Approach to Electrodermal Activity Processing. *IEEE Trans. Biomed. Eng.* **2016**, *63*, 797–804. [CrossRef]
43. Kappeler-Setz, C. *Multimodal Emotion and Stress Recognition*; ETH Zurich: Zurich, Switzerland, 2012; pp. 20–26.
44. Kim, H.G.; Cheon, E.J.; Bai, D.S.; Lee, Y.H.; Koo, B.H. Stress and heart rate variability: A meta-analysis and review of the literature. *Psychiatry Investig.* **2018**, *15*, 235. [CrossRef]
45. MATLAB. 9.7.0.1190202 (R2019b); The MathWorks Inc.: Natick, MA, USA, 2018.
46. Stress Response. Available online: https://www.anxietycentre.com/anxiety/stress-response.shtml (accessed on 25 February 2020).
47. Tarvainen, M.P.; Niskanen, J.P.; Lipponen, J.A.; Ranta-aho, P.O.; Karjalainen, P.A. Kubios HRV—A Software for Advanced Heart Rate Variability Analysis. In Proceedings of the 4th European Conference of the International Federation for Medical and Biological Engineering, Antwerp, Belgium, 23–27 November 2008; Vander Sloten, J.; Verdonck, P.; Nyssen, M.; Haueisen, J., Eds.; Springer: Berlin/Heidelberg, Germany, 2009; pp. 1022–1025.

48. Cinaz, B.; Arnrich, B.; Marca, R.; Tröster, G. Monitoring of Mental Workload Levels During an Everyday Life Office-work Scenario. *Pers. Ubiquitous Comput.* **2013**, *17*, 229–239. [CrossRef]
49. Alberdi, A.; Aztiria, A.; Basarab, A. Towards an automatic early stress recognition system for office environments based on multimodal measurements: A review. *J. Biomed. Inform.* **2016**, *59*, 49–75. [CrossRef]
50. Greene, S.; Thapliyal, H.; Caban-Holt, A. A Survey of Affective Computing for Stress Detection: Evaluating technologies in stress detection for better health. *IEEE Consum. Electron. Mag.* **2016**, *5*, 44–56. [CrossRef]
51. Castellano, G.; Villalba, S.D.; Camurri, A. Recognising human emotions from body movement and gesture dynamics. In Proceedings of the International Conference on Affective Computing and Intelligent Interaction, Lisbon, Portugal, 12–14 September 2007; pp. 71–82.
52. Melzer, A.; Shafir, T.; Tsachor, R.P. How Do We Recognize Emotion From Movement? Specific Motor Components Contribute to the Recognition of Each Emotion. *Front. Psychol.* **2019**, *10*, 1389. [CrossRef]
53. Tang, T.B.; Yeo, L.W.; Lau, D.J.H. Activity awareness can improve continuous stress detection in galvanic skin response. In Proceedings of the IEEE SENSORS 2014, Valencia, Spain, 2–5 November 2014; pp. 1980–1983.
54. Eibe, F.; Hall, M.; Witten, I. *The WEKA Workbench. Online Appendix for "Data Mining: Practical Machine Learning Tools and Techniques"*; Morgan Kaufmann: Burlington, MA, USA, 2016.
55. Zhang, W.; Ramezani, R.; Naeim, A. WOTBoost: Weighted Oversampling Technique in Boosting for imbalanced learning. *arXiv* **2019**, arXiv:1910.07892.
56. Holmes, G.; Donkin, A.; Witten, I.H. WEKA: A machine learning workbench. In Proceedings of the ANZIIS'94—Australian New Zealnd Intelligent Information Systems Conference, Brisbane, Australia, 29 November–2 December 1994; pp. 357–361.
57. Hart, S.G. *NASA Task Load Index (TLX)*; Paper and Pencil Package; NASA Ames Research Center: Mountain View, CA, USA, 1986; Volume 1.0.
58. Glasman, L.R.; Albarracin, D. Forming attitudes that predict future behavior: A meta-analysis of the attitude-behavior relation. *Psychol. Bull.* **2006**, *132*, 778. [CrossRef]

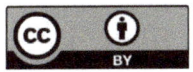

© 2020 by the authors. Licensee MDPI, Basel, Switzerland. This article is an open access article distributed under the terms and conditions of the Creative Commons Attribution (CC BY) license (http://creativecommons.org/licenses/by/4.0/).

MDPI
St. Alban-Anlage 66
4052 Basel
Switzerland
Tel. +41 61 683 77 34
Fax +41 61 302 89 18
www.mdpi.com

Healthcare Editorial Office
E-mail: healthcare@mdpi.com
www.mdpi.com/journal/healthcare

www.ingramcontent.com/pod-product-compliance
Lightning Source LLC
LaVergne TN
LVHW070547100526
838202LV00012B/402